Federico Pea

Pharmacokinetics in Everyday Clinical Practice

SEEd

© **SEE*d* srl**
Via Magenta, 35 – 10128 Torino (Italy)
Tel. +39.011.566.02.58
www.edizioniseed.it
info@edizioniseed.it

ISBN 978-88-9741-917-4

Although the information about medication given in this book has been carefully checked, the author and publisher accept no liability for the accuracy of this information. In every individual case the user must check such information by consulting the relevant literature.

TABLE OF CONTENTS

INTRODUCTION

Pharmacokinetics is a branch of pharmacology that studies the velocity of the processes that determine the course of the plasma concentration of a drug. By applying a series of mathematical models, it enables to quantitatively describe the movement of a drug in the body over time. This is the result of the various phases that occur after administration of a drug, i.e., absorp-

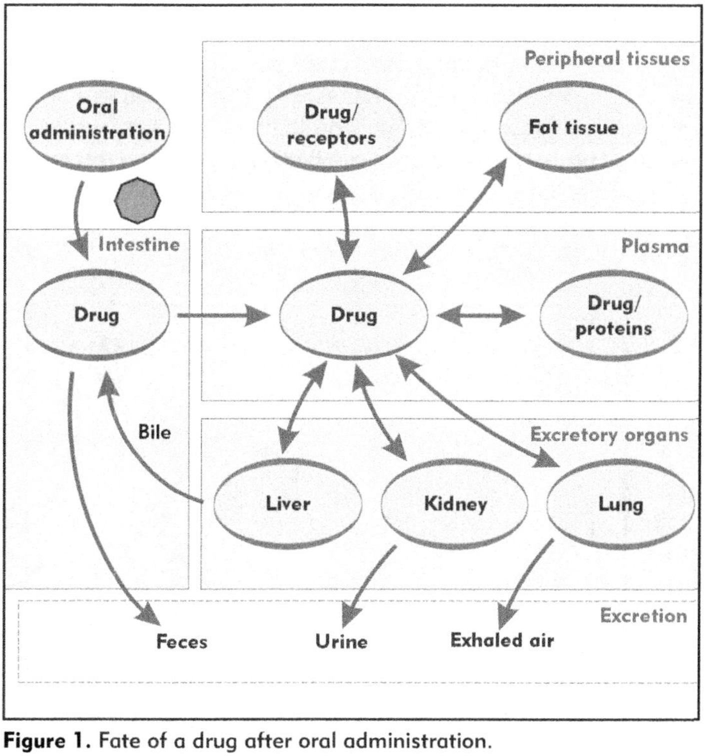

Figure 1. Fate of a drug after oral administration.

tion, distribution, metabolism and excretion. Knowing the "fate" of a drug in the body is the prerequisite for defining the most appropriate dosing regimen, in terms of amount and frequency of administration, in order to obtain the desired therapeutic effect. In fact, the therapeutic effect of a drug depends on the achievement of effective concentrations in target tissues. As an example, we can imagine what might be the fate of a drug after oral administration (Figure 1).

After being ingested, and having reached the gastrointestinal system, the drug, if it has suitable physicochemical characteristics, is absorbed and eventually enters the bloodstream. At this level, the drug binds to plasma proteins (in most cases with albumin), to a different degree depending on the circumstances, and then is distributed to various organs and tissues. Only the free moiety of the drug is "biologically active," which means that only the unbound fraction can diffuse out of the bloodstream to be distributed through the tissues. After this, in order to be eliminated, the drug must pass through the emunctory organs, in which it may or may not undergo biotransformation (metabolism), and is then excreted, as appropriate, by the kidney, or gut, or via other minor pathways (e.g., exhaled air, sweat, etc.).

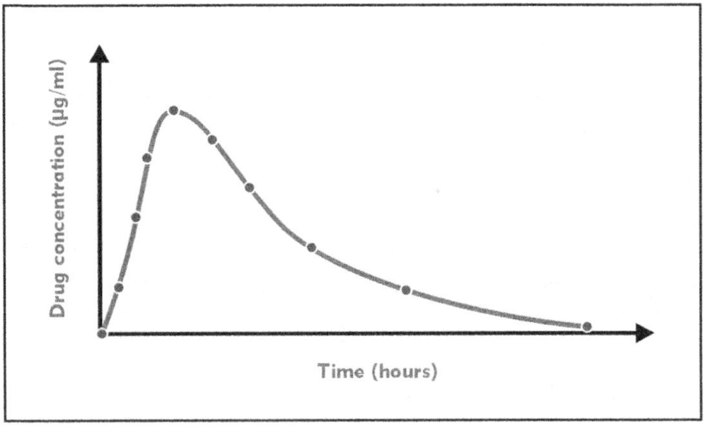

Figure 2. Plasma concentration versus time curve.

In this scenario, plasma essentially represents the mean by which the drug is conveyed to the various districts within the body. For this reason, knowing the plasma concentration profile of a drug in relation to the time after its administration can be a useful tool for understanding its pharmacokinetic behavior in the body (Figure 2).
The aim of this publication is not to define the strict mathematical rules that are the basis for pharmacokinetic studies conducted by experts, but to help all physicians to become familiar with some concepts that will enable them to apply the principles of pharmacokinetics in the daily management of their patients' treatments. Therefore, unlike in specialized texts, the use of mathematical formulas will be minimal, serving only to help physicians to understand these concepts.

1 PHARMACOKINETICS AND TERMINOLOGY

The usefulness of pharmacokinetics in the daily management of therapy can be more easily understood by defining and explaining the major pharmacokinetic parameters, as summarized in Table I.

1.1 Oral Bioavailability (F_{os})

The bioavailability of a drug is defined as **the fraction of a drug (F) which, after administration by a route different from the intravenous one, reaches the systemic circulation in unchanged form (i.e., therapeutically active form), and the rapidity with which it does so**. The pharmacokinetic parameter that best defines F is represented by the area under the plasma concentration-time curve (AUC), as shown in Figure 3.

Pharmacokinetic parameter	Abbreviation
Oral bioavailability	F_{os}
Volume of distribution	V_d
Plasma clearance	CL
Plasma elimination half-life	$t_{1/2}$
Area under the plasma concentration versus time curve	AUC
Steady state plasma concentration	C_{ss}
Loading dose	LD
Maintenance dose	MD

Table I. Major pharmacokinetic parameters.

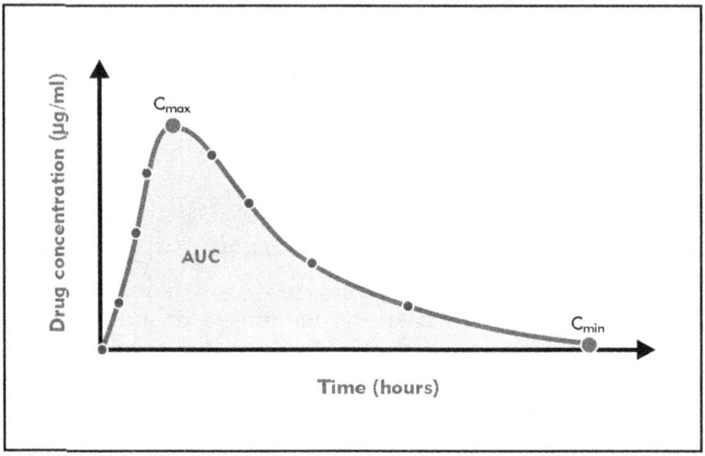

Figure 3. Plasma concentration-time curve.
C_{max} = maximum concentration; C_{min} = minimum or pre-dose concentration

The AUC may be defined as **a quantitative parameter of systemic drug exposure**, because it is informative on the total amount of drug which is present in the body throughout the day (AUC_{24h}). In order to properly evaluate the absolute F of a drug after oral administration (F_{os}), it is necessary to compare the AUC obtained after this route of administration (AUC_{os}) with the reference one, i.e., that obtained after administration of a single intravenous dose (AUC_{iv}). In fact, AUC_{iv} has by definition an F of 100% since the drug administered intravenously enters directly into the bloodstream with no need of absorption. To properly assess $F_{os,}$ a specific method is used, in which a single dose of the drug is administered by the two routes – at two subsequent times to the same subjects (Figure 4): first, by one route (e.g., IV), collecting a series of blood samples over time in order to assess AUC_{iv}; subsequently, after a period of time long enough to allow the complete elimination of the drug (washout), the same dose of the drug is administered by the other route (e.g., orally), and finally the AUC_{os} is estimated through serial blood collection.

$$F_{os} = \frac{AUC_{os} \times 100}{AUC_{iv}}$$

The minimum and maximum values of F_{os} are 0 and 100%, respectively, when the drug does not reach the systemic circulation (because it is unabsorbable by this route of administration, as for example occur for water-soluble drugs such as beta-lactam antibiotics, aminoglycosides and glycopeptides), or when it reaches it *in toto* as unchanged moiety (e.g., when it is completely absorbed without undergoing any change).
Intermediate values of F_{os} indicate that only part of the drug administered orally is able to reach the systemic circulation in active form. This may be the consequence of an only partial absorption at the gastrointestinal level, or of partial presystemic metabolic biotransformation that may occur during the passage through the gut wall and/or the portal circulation and the liver (the so-called **first-pass effect**). In fact, the oral absorption of

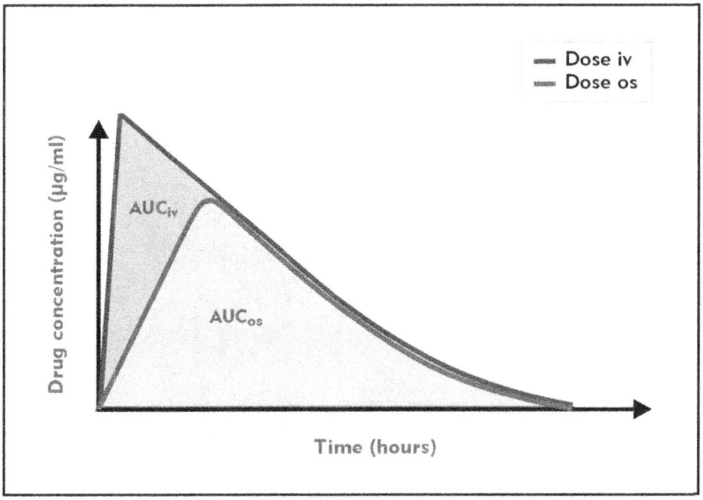

Figure 4. Calculation of oral bioavailability of a drug. F_{os} can be calculated directly from the ratio of the two AUCs, namely: $(AUC_{os} \times 100)/AUC_{iv}$.

a drug depends mainly on its physicochemical properties, which determine whether or not it can freely cross the plasma membrane of eukaryotic cells (in this case the intestinal wall). Only

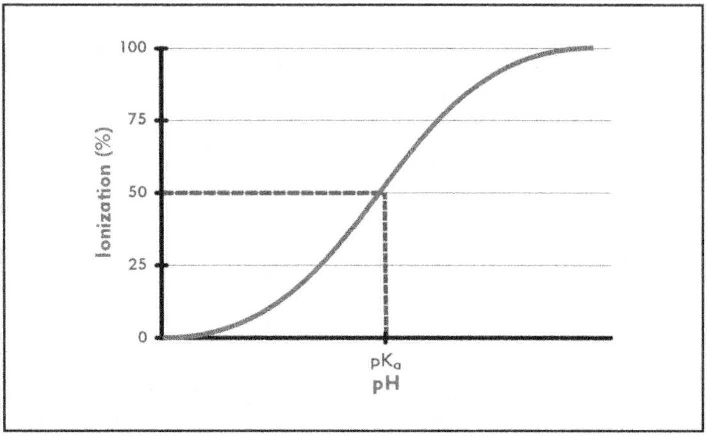

Figure 5. Dissociation curve of weak acids, that are better absorbed in the stomach.

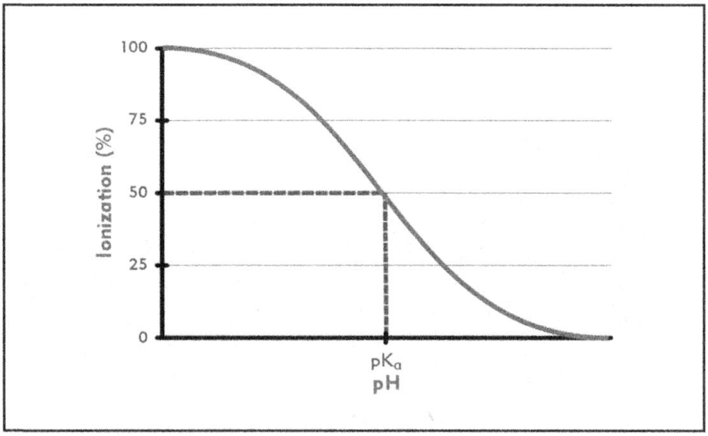

Figure 6. Dissociation curve of weak bases, that are better absorbed in the intestine.

lipid soluble drugs, in fact, are able to cross cell membranes through a process of passive diffusion according to a concentration gradient (from the more concentrated environment to the less concentrated one).
In this respect, it should be noted that most of the drugs are weak electrolytes: that is to say, they are substances that are in equilibrium between a dissociated form and an undissociated one, on the basis of their dissociation constant (pK_a = pH value at which the drug is for 50% in the dissociated form and for the other 50% in the undissociated one) and of the pH value of the environment. Since only the undissociated fraction of a weak electrolyte is sufficiently liposoluble to be absorbed by passive diffusion, it follows that the more the value of the pK_a of the drug will be similar to the pH of the gastrointestinal tract, the larger the absorbed amount will be.
Consequently, weak acids are more undissociated at acidic pH (Figure 5) and are therefore better absorbed in the stomach, whereas weak bases are more undissociated at alkaline pH (Figure 6) and are therefore better absorbed in the intestine.

1.1.1 | Clinical Meaning of F_{os}

The clinical usefulness of knowing the F_{os} of a drug is to be able to determine the appropriateness of a dosing regimen when treatment is performed **sequentially**.
Sequential therapy means the opportunity of treating patients with the same drug sequentially by different routes of administration (usually before by IV and subsequently per os), according to the severity of the disease, but with the intent of ensuring equal therapeutic efficacy. In this regard, it is clear which is the purpose of knowing the F_{os} of a drug: indeed, it is a key factor in defining which dose is to be used orally in order to obtain equal exposure (AUC), and therefore equal efficacy, in comparison with the intravenous one (Figure 7).
For example, if AUC_{os} is equal to AUC_{iv}, the same dose is to be used orally; but if AUC_{os} is only 25% of AUC_{iv}, the oral dosage must be four times higher than the intravenous one.

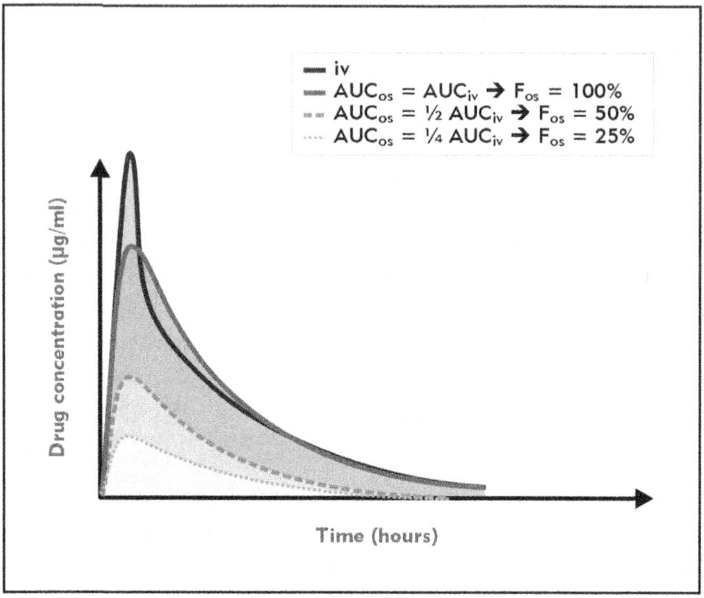

Figure 7. Calculation of dosage equivalence.

Such considerations help to explain why for some drugs the oral doses may be several folds higher than those used intravenously (e.g., ganciclovir).

1.2 Apparent Volume of Distribution (V_d)

The apparent volume of distribution of a drug (V_d) corresponds to a fictitious value, which is defined as **the volume that the drug would occupy in the body if it had in all the body districts the same concentration that it has in plasma at time 0 after administration by intravenous bolus injection**.
This definition seems particularly complex; indeed, it can be more easily understood if it is analyzed in detail from a clinical pharmaocological point of view. First, the choice of intravenous bolus administration of the drug for the study of V_d is intended

	Drug A	Drug B
Dose (mg)	100	100
C_{p0} (mg/l)	10	0.1
V_d (l) = D/C_{p0}	10	1,000

Table II. Volume of distribution (V_d) of a drug on the basis of plasma concentration at time 0 (C_{p0}).

to limit the pharmacokinetic event, thus allowing only the assessment of the period of distribution. In fact, the use of intravenous administration allows to avoid the appearance of the phase which comes before the distribution when other routes of administration are used, namely absorption; while the speed of the bolus administration, followed by immediate sampling, allows that the plasma concentration measured at time 0 is the result solely of the distribution, because the elimination process has not yet begun. On the basis of this definition the formula is:

$$V_d = \frac{D}{C_{p0}}$$

where D is the administered dose of the drug and C_{p0} is the plasma concentration measured at the end of the IV bolus. On this basis, it is clear that, under the same administered dose (i.e. 100 mg), the lower the C_{p0} resulted, the higher the V_d of the drug will be (Table II).

1.2.1 Clinical Meaning of V_d

From a clinical point of view, the usefulness of V_d is essentially that of making understandable where the drug is compartmentalized and to what extent it accumulates in tissues.

In this respect, it becomes crucial to consider the different "hydric" compartments of the body (Figure 8). These are represented by the plasma, the interstitial fluids, and the intracellular fluids. If we imagine a subject weighing about 70 kg, his/her total body water, which is about 38-44 liters, is divided as follows:

- 3 l in plasma;
- 10-13 l in interstitial fluids;
- 25-28 l in intracellular fluids.

In relation to the distribution of a drug in these compartments, three different cases are possible.

The first case is that of a drug that, after being administered intravenously, cannot exit the bloodstream; for example, as a consequence of its high molecular weight, similar to or greater than that of plasma protein (30,000 D), which does not allow it to pass through the "pores" of fenestrated capillaries. This drug will therefore have a V_d similar to that of plasma (approximately 3 l). This is the case, for example, of the so-called "plasma substitutes" or "plasma expanders," such as crystalloids and colloids, whose function is essentially oncotic, that is to say, to maintain adequate blood volume, such as in polytrauma patients.

The second situation is that of those drugs which are able to distribute, not only in plasma, but even in the interstitial fluid of

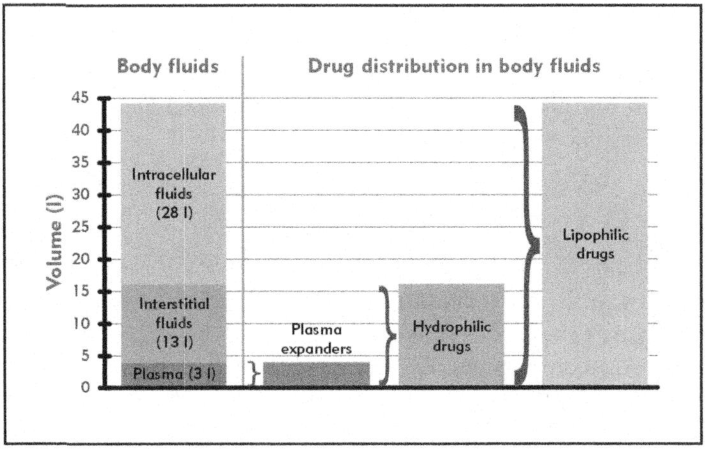

Figure 8. Body water compartments.

tissues, but are unable to penetrate intracellularly. These drugs will have a V_d that is more or less equal to that resulting from the sum of the two extracellular compartments, about 13-16 l. This is the case of many antibiotics such as beta-lactams, aminoglycosides and glycopeptides, which, being hydrophilic substances, are unable of passively diffuse through the plasmatic membrane of the eukaryotic cells, thus remaining localized only outside the cells.

On the other hand, it must be taken into account that the majority of pathogenic bacteria have an extracellular localization, that is the bloodstream and/or the interstitium of tissues. This fact allows to explain, from a pharmacokinetic point of view, why these antibiotics are effective in treating most of the bacterial infections.

The third case is that of a drug which, according to some peculiar physicochemical properties, such as lipophilicity and low molecular weight, is able to freely diffuse (by passive diffusion according to the concentration gradient) in the different body districts. This drug has a V_d which is similar to the total body water volume, namely about 40 l.

Nevertheless, some drugs may have V_d which can be of the order of several hundreds or even thousands of liters. This is the case, for example, of digoxin, which has a V_d of about 400 liters, or of chloroquine, whose V_d is of about 14,000 l.

Obviously, these are not real values, but fictitious ones, corresponding, as mentioned above, to the **volume that the drug would occupy in the body if it had in all body districts the same concentration that it has in plasma at time 0 after administration by intravenous bolus injection**. These values indicate that these drugs are mainly segregated within cells, which therefore act as reservoirs.

This appears to be a consequence of the fact that some drugs may significantly bind, often reversibly, to some cellular structures, usually proteins, so that their intracellular concentrations can be several folds higher than the extracellular ones.

In pharmacokinetic studies V_d is usually expressed, irrespective of body weight, in l/kg. Referring to the aforementioned examples, this value can be obtained by dividing the reported V_d by the weight of the subject (70 kg). Simplistically, we might say that:

- drugs with $V_d < 0.7$-1 l/kg are distributed exclusively in the extracellular compartment;
- drugs with $V_d > 1$ l/kg are distributed also in the intracellular compartment.

The V_d of a drug is also influenced by the extent of plasma protein binding.

In fact, considering that under physiological conditions plasma proteins do not exit the bloodstream, it is clear that the amount of the drug bound to them cannot distribute.

This concept also allows to explain an axiom frequently reported in pharmacology textbooks: **only the amount of the free drug is biologically active**.

In fact, this means that only the proportion of the free drug, by diffusing out of the bloodstream according to the pharmacokinetic principles, is able to reach its site of action at the tissue level, thus interacting with the receptors.

From these considerations it is obvious that V_d is also a relevant factor conditioning the time that a drug remains in the body.

In fact, as showed later, it correlates directly to the plasma elimination half-life ($t_{1/2}$), since the more the drug is segregated into different organs and tissues, the greater will be the time required for it to come back into the bloodstream and then to reach the emuntory organs to be eliminated.

1.3 Plasma Clearance (CL)

The plasma clearance of a drug (CL) is defined as **the volume of plasma that is cleared by the drug in the unit of time**.

Therefore it is measured in units of flow and can be expressed, for example, in liters per hour (l/h) or milliliters per minute (ml/min).

Obviously, it is possible to switch between the two modes of expression: to pass from liters per hour to milliliters per minute, the result has to be multiplied by 1,000 and divided by 60; whereas to do the opposite, result has to be divided by 1,000 and multiplied by 60. For example, a CL of 0.6 l/h is equivalent to a value of 10 ml/min.

The total body CL (CL_t) is the result of the elimination of the drug through all the emuntory organs. These are mainly the liver and/or the kidneys, although sometimes there are secondary routes of elimination, such as exhaled air in the case of drugs that are gas and/or in the volatile state.

Very often the hydrophilic drugs (for example, many antibiotics), due to their physicochemical characteristics, are eliminated by the kidneys as unchanged drug, that is in the same form as they were introduced into the body, without any rearrangement in their structure. Therefore, plasma claerance of some drugs depends mainly on the kidney (renal clearance, CL_r).

In contrast, lipophilic drugs often require one or more processes of metabolism (**biotransformation**) before being eliminated from the body, and this function depends mainly by the liver (Table III).

Therefore, for many lipophilic drugs, clearance is mainly hepatic (CL_h).

In general, the greater the degree of lipophilicity of the drug is, the greater the need for biotransformation will be. It should be taken into consideration that highly lipophilic drugs may require

Nonsynthetic reactions (phase I)	• Oxidative deamination • Hydrolysis (esters, amides, glycosides) • Oxidations • Reductions
Synthetic reactions (phase II)	• Alkylation: transfer of methyl radicals • Acylation: introduction of acetyl radicals • Conjugations (by transferases): · With glucuronic acid · With sulfuric acid · With aminoacids

Table III. Main processes of drug biotransformation.

several metabolic processes, of different types and in sequence, in order to make them completely eliminable from the body.
In fact, the main purpose of the metabolism is to produce metabolites that are more hydrophilic than the parent drug, and thus more easily eliminable.
This is the consequence of the fact that, generally speaking, when a lipophilic drug comes into pre-urine after glomerular filtration in the kidney, it is normally reabsorbed in tubules according to the principles of passive diffusion, and obviously this reabsorption slows its elimination.
A particular example of this is offered by diazepam. This benzodiazepine undergoes various processes of metabolism (demethylation, hydroxylation and conjugation); and it is noteworthy that some of its intermediate metabolites are pharmaco-

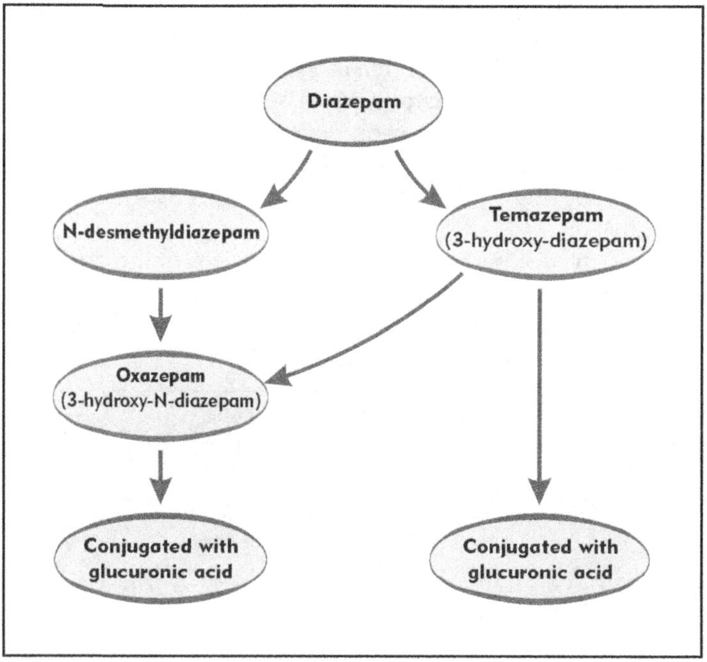

Figure 9. Diazepam and its metabolites.

E	Examples of drugs	F_{os} (%)
Drugs with high E (> 60%)	Fluvastatin, imipramine, isosorbide dinitrate, lovastatin, morphine, nitroglycerin, sertraline	< 40
Drugs with intermediate E (30-60%)	Amiodarone, amitriptyline, atorvastatin, clomipramine, codeine, erythromycin, pravastatin, simvastatin	40-70
Drugs with low E (< 30%)	Clarithromycin, clofibrate, gemfibrozil, prednisolone, tolbutamide	> 70

Table IV. **Classification of drugs in relation to the degree of hepatic extraction (E) and their bioavailability after oral administration (F_{os}).**

logically active, so that they are themselves used routinary as benzodiazepines in therapy (e.g., desmethyldiazepam, oxazepam, and temazepam) (Figure 9).

According to the rapidity and to the way by which they are extracted from the liver—according to their extraction index (E)—drugs can be classified into three groups (Table IV).

The so-called drugs at high hepatic extraction, after oral administration, usually undergo to extraction rate of ≥ 60% during the "first pass" through the liver, and their CL is mainly dependent on hepatic blood flow. This phenomenon, which is described as the "first-pass effect", results in a consistent reduction of the bioavailable moiety. Therefore, drugs with high E, under normal conditions have F_{os} ≤ 40% and high CL_h.

The so-called drugs at intermediate hepatic extraction (30-60%) have a CL dependent both on the hepatic blood flow and on the intrinsic hepatocyte activity, i.e., on the amount of the enzymatic activity. In general, their F_{os} is higher and their CL_h is lower than those observed for drugs with high hepatic extraction.

The so-called drugs at low hepatic extraction (< 30%) are poorly metabolized during the first pass through the liver and their CL_h depends more on the intrinsic activity of hepatocytes, than on the hepatic blood flow.

Under normal conditions, their F_{os} is > 70% and their CL_h more moderate.

1.3.1 | Clinical Meaning of CL

According to the definition of CL (**volume of plasma cleared per unit of time**) it is clear that, under physiological conditions, the maximum value of CL for a given drug will necessarily correspond to the respective plasma flows of each emunctory organ. Therefore, under physiological conditions, the maximum CL_r can correspond to the value of renal plasma flow (650 ml/min) and the maximum CL_h can correspond to the value of hepatic blood flow (1,500 ml/min).
In practice, this means that when a drug has a CL_t higher than 650 ml/min, it is certainly eliminated not only by the renal route. In fact, when assessing the role that the kidney may play in drug elimination of a (CL_r), several cases may occur (Table V).
In the kidneys a drug may undergo three types of rearrangements: glomerular filtration, tubular secretion and active tubular reabsorption. The glomerular filtration is a process to which all drugs are subjected. In fact, the molecular weight of most drugs is far below the glomerular filtration cut-off (30,000-60,000 D), corresponding to the molecular weight of plasma proteins.

CL_r (ml/min)	Clinical meaning
0	Drug filtered through the glomerulus, but completely reabsorbed in the tubules → often very lipophilic drug
0.1-120	Drug filtered through the glomerulus, but partially reabsorbed in the tubules
120	Drug filtered through the glomerulus, which is neither reabsorbed nor secreted in the tubules → often hydrophilic drug
120-650	Drug filtered through the glomerulus and partially secreted in the tubules
650	Drug filtered through the glomerulus and completely secreted in the tubules

Table V. Clinical significance of renal clearance (CL_r) under physiological conditions.

Therefore, under physiological conditions, if the CL_r value is equal to 0 ml/min, the plasma that passes through the kidney is not cleared from that drug because the drug, after being filtered in the glomeruli, is completely reabsorbed by passive diffusion in the tubules. This is usually the case of many highly lipophilic drugs which, due to this reason, need to be metabolized to become more hydrophilic and to be eliminated from the body. If the CL_r value is 120 ml/min, i.e., equal to the physiological value of glomerular filtration rate, it is likely that, after being filtered in the glomeruli, the drug will not undergo any further rearrangement in the tubules, being neither actively secreted nor reabsorbed.
If the value is equal to 650 ml/min, this means that the plasma passing through the kidney is completely cleared from the drug in question, since the drug, other than being filtered through the glomeruli, has been actively secreted in the tubules.
Of course, intermediate CL_r values correspond to intermediate situations (see Table V). In particular, it should also be noted that plasma protein binding is a factor that slows down drug elimination, since only the free moiety can be eliminated from plasma. When a drug is mainly eliminated through hepatic biotransformation, CL_h values are often higher than 650-700 ml/min, till reaching a maximum value which may be equal to the hepatic blood flow.

1.4 Area Under the Plasma Concentration-time Curve (AUC)

Plasma drug exposure may be expressed quantitatively in terms of AUC. This is the result of the balance between **input**, in terms of dose, and **output**, in terms of CL, and when the drug is administered intravenously, it is expressed by the following formula (Figure 10):

$$AUC_{iv} = \frac{dose}{CL}$$

When the drug is administered orally, its F_{os} must be taken into account in this formula, as follows:

$$AUC_{os} = \frac{dose \times F_{os}}{CL}$$

If the CL of a drug remains constant, this means that the exposure increases in direct proportion to the dose, that is in an absolutely predictable manner. This is what happens when the CL of the drug is independent from the dose, i.e., when the kinetic process is defined as of **first order** or dose-independent. This feature is typical of drugs that are primarily eliminated by the kidney, since glomerular filtration is a process that does not come to saturation, and in these circumstances the elimination rate increases directly with increasing concentration ($v = k \times C$). In the case of drugs that are eliminated by the liver it is necessary to bear in mind that in the processes of biotransformation there is a saturation limit which, based on the Michaelis-Menten equation, is represented by the maximum velocity (v_{max}) at which the enzyme responsible for this function can work in the presence of an excess of substrate.

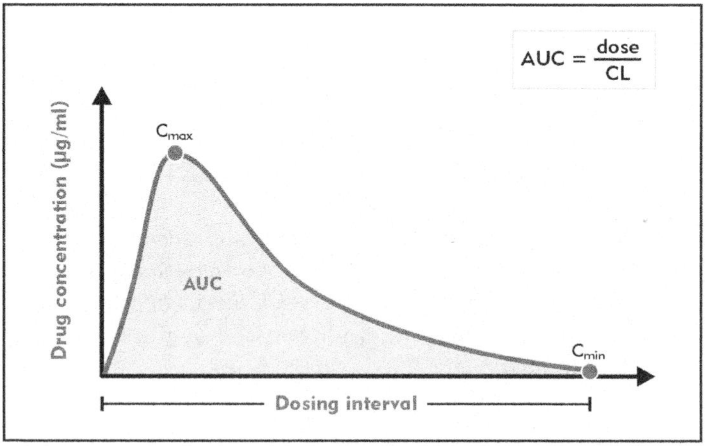

Figure 10. Plasmatic exposure to the drug and clearance.

Indeed, several drugs that we use in daily clinical practice, despite having a predominantly hepatic CL, follow a dose-independent kinetics, similarly to what happens for those cleared by glomerular filtration, because the plasma concentrations achieved with the usual therapeutic doses are lower than those needed to saturate the enzyme kinetics.
However, there are some exceptions: for example, phenytoin, already at therapeutic doses, may exhibit a zero order kinetics, or dose-dependent, since there is a saturation of metabolic processes, so that the elimination rate cannot grow further with increasing concentration (v = k). This means that, unlike in the 1st order kinetics, the CL is not a typical constant of the drug but can vary with dose, so that when increasing the dose, drug exposure does not increase linearly in a predictable manner, but much higher in an unpredictable manner.
In clinical practice some specific situations may cause the saturation of the elimination process of a drug.
For example in the case of drugs eliminated by the liver, this may occur during polytherapy as a result of peculiar drug-drug pharmacokinetic interactions polytherapy, especially when are added drugs that may inhibit the enzyme activity, the so-called enzymatic inhibitors. This topic will be specifically discussed in chapter 2, which is dedicated to pharmacokinetic interactions.

1.4.1 | Clinical Meaning of AUC

The AUC could be defined as a parameter of **quantitative exposure** to a drug. In other words, it is expression of how much drug is present in the body throughout the day, and this is helpful in understanding how much drug should be administered daily in order to maintain a therapeutically effective exposure over time. As aforementioned, in the same subject the AUC varies when the CL changes and, therefore in specific pathophysiological conditions the AUC can significantly change as a consequence of changes in the function of the emuntory organs.
It must also be considered that the AUC is not a **qualitative** parameter, and this means that it is not expression of how the

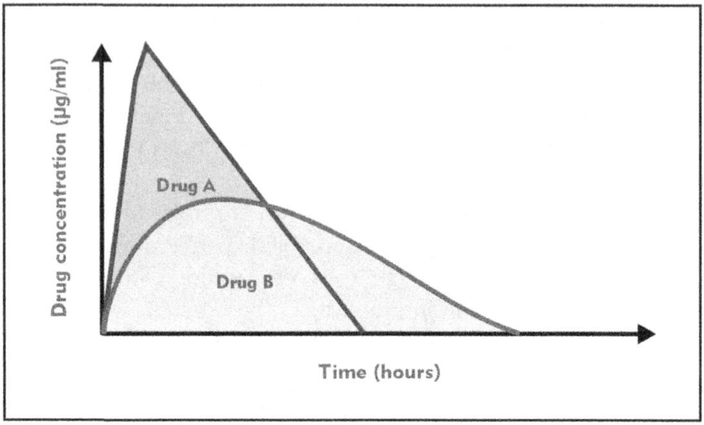

Figure 11. AUC and exposure profiles.

drug is present in the body over time. In fact, two drugs, although having the same value of AUC, may exhibit completely different exposure profiles in the body, as reported for drugs A and B in the example shown in Figure 11. This is obviously the result of completely different pharmacokinetic behaviors (in fact, it is not surprising that geometric figures with different shapes can have the same area value).

1.5 Plasma Elimination Half-life ($t_{1/2}$)

Considering that V_d and CL are the two main parameters that may independently affect the kinetic behavior of a drug in the body, it is understandable why the drug elimination time is a function of both of these parameters. In fact, the plasma elimination half-life ($t_{1/2}$), that is the **time required for the amount of a substance to decrease by a half**, can be calculated using the following formula:

$$t_{1/2} = \frac{0.693 \times V_d}{CL}$$

This means that the $t_{1/2}$ of a drug will be longer:

- The higher its V_d is, i.e., the larger its accumulation within the intracellular space of tissues is.
- The lower its CL is, i.e., the lower the plasma volume purified by the drug in the unit of time is.

1.5.1 | Clinical Meaning of $t_{1/2}$

The $t_{1/2}$ of a drug is the main pharmacokinetic parameter that should be taken into consideration in order to choose an appropriate dosing regimen, in particular in relation to the frequency of daily administration. This is due to the fact that the time required for complete removal of a drug from the body after a single dose is equal to 4-5 folds its $t_{1/2,}$ and in most cases (1st order kinetics) this time is independent from the administered dose and from the concentrations achieved in the body. It derives from this axiom that drugs with very short $t_{1/2}$ (shorter than 1-2 hours) should be administered frequently, every 4-6 hours, in order to allow the continuous maintenance of therapeutically effective concentrations. This concept becomes even more compelling in the case of drugs with a $t_{1/2}$ of only few minutes, as in the case of certain hormones and/or neuromodulators, such as dopamine and/or oxytocin. Therefore, in these cases administering the drug by continuous intravenous infusion is the only way to maintain therapeutically effective concentrations over time. On the other hand, for drugs with prolonged $t_{1/2}$ (longer than 12-24 hours), a single daily dosing, or even an alternate-day dosing may suffice. In general, therefore, the shorter the drug $t_{1/2}$ is, the closer the administration time should be.In the presence of peculiar pathophysiological conditions, it becomes clear that in a given patient the $t_{1/2}$ of a specific drug may undergo significant changes as a consequence of diseases and/or of iatrogenic situations which may significantly affect its V_d and/or its CL.

1.6 Steady State Plasma Concentration (C_{ss})

Steady state plasma concentration (C_{ss}) can be defined as **the plasma concentration reached by a drug in the body at the time a "steady state" has been achieved, and then maintained. This happens when the rate of drug administration and that of drug elimination becomes equal and there is stable equilibrium between the "drug inputs," i.e., the administered doses, and the " drug outputs," i.e., the amount eliminated by the excretory organs**.

Once a therapy with multiple doses of a drug has been started, the time required to reach the steady state is equal to 4-5 times its $t_{1/2}$.

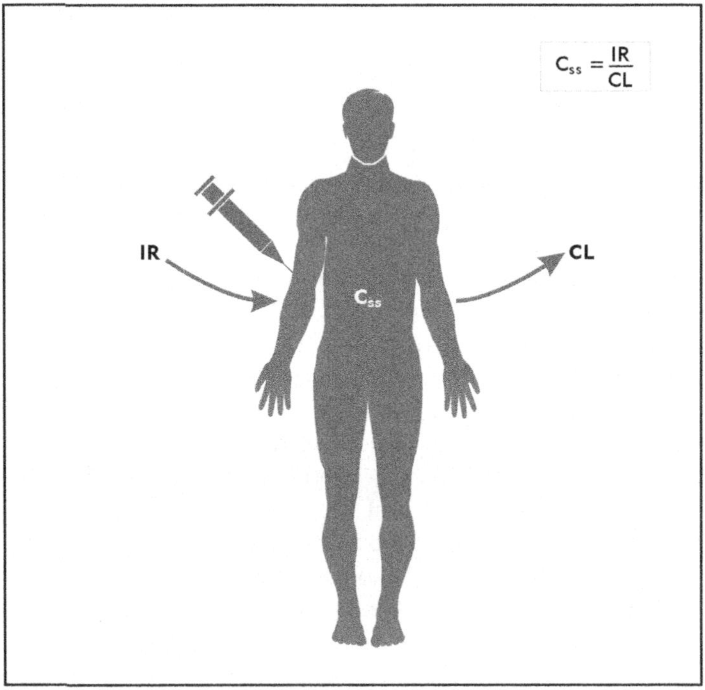

Figure 12. C_{ss} and continuous intravenous infusion.

It follows therefore that, while for drugs with short $t_{1/2}$ the steady state is reached even within few hours after starting therapy, for drugs with long $t_{1/2}$ it will take several days or even weeks before they can achieve the steady state. The C_{ss} will be really constant only if the drug is administered by continuous intravenous infusion, since in such circumstances the amount of drug that has been eliminated through the excretory organs is replaced in real time, second by second:

$$C_{ss} = \frac{IR}{CL}$$

where IR is the infusion rate of the drug (Figure 12).
In all other situations where intermittent therapy is performed, of course, concentrations fluctuate between a minimum and a maximum depending on the time between doses, regardless of

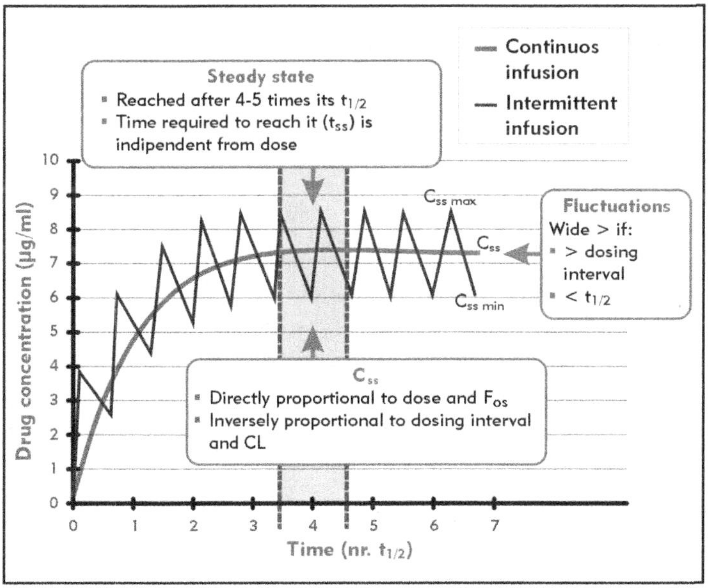

Figure 13. Steady state concentration (C_{ss}) in the case of therapy with intermittent dosing.

the route of administration, so that there will be a $C_{ss\ min}$ and a $C_{ss\ max}$ (Figure 13).
In any case, such fluctuations between maximum and minimum steady values will remain constant only if the time interval between doses is kept constant, i.e., if the doses are equally distributed throughout the day and always administered at the same hour (e.g., if the posology of a drug is 3 times daily, the dose should be administered every 8 hours).

1.6.1 | Clinical Meaning of C_{ss}

C_{ss} generally corresponds to the effective concentrations that must be achieved and then maintained in the body during drug therapy.
From this consideration it appears that, whereas for drugs with short $t_{1/2}$ the therapeutic efficacy may onset just at the beginning of therapy, for drugs with long $t_{1/2}$ a considerable period of latency may elapse before the appearance of the therapeutic effect linked to the achievement of C_{ss}. For example, with regard to drugs such as digoxin or tricyclic antidepressants which have long $t_{1/2}$, those therapies started with standard doses are characterized by a latency of several days before the appearance of a good therapeutic effect.
Of note, in certain circumstances and/or for certain drugs with long $t_{1/2}$, it may be necessary to achieve therapeutically effective concentrations since the beginning of therapy, and such concentrations should obviously be as high as those observed at the steady state. This can be achieved by administering the so-called loading dose (LD).

1.7 Loading Dose (LD)

The LD is the dose of medication always larger than the subsequent doses that is administered at the beginning of therapy with the purpose of filling rapidly the V_d occupied by the drug,

thus enabling the early achievement of therapeutically effective concentrations at its site of action.
LD can be easily calculated using the following formula:

$$LD = V_d \times C_{target}$$

where C_{target} is the target concentration that must be rapidly achieved.
From this definition some important considerations can be deduced:

- LD is essential to obtain a rapid therapeutic response for drugs with long $t_{1/2}$, because if not administered, the period of latency until the onset of effects may be incompatible with a prompt therapeutic response. This can be a relevant issue in some specific cases: for example, for the antibiotic therapy with teicoplanin, for the heart failure therapy with digoxin in the intensive care setting or for the treatment of status epilepticus with phenobarbital.
- If the LD is necessary, it must be administered to all of the patients, regardless of the functionality of the excretory organs (e.g., kidney and/or liver), since it depends solely on the V_d of the drug and therefore only on the "body weight" of the patient and not on the CL, that is on the functionality of its excretory organs.

1.8 Maintenance Dose (MD)

The literal definition of the so-called maintenance dose (MD) highlights that the primary purpose of this dose is to allow the maintenance of therapeutically effective concentrations that have been previously achieved with the LD.
Indeed, in several cases, the short $t_{1/2}$ of the used drug allows the achievement of the C_{ss} followed by the full therapeutic effect within a relatively short period of time, so that administration of an LD is not essential.

For example, in the case of drugs with $t_{1/2} < 6$ hours, C_{ss} is reached already within the first day of therapy. For this reason, in the dosing regimens of drugs with medium-short $t_{1/2}$ often there is no distinction between the LD and the MD; that is to say, the administered dose is always the same regardless of whether you are at the beginning of therapy or during its continuation. On the other hand, as already mentioned in the previous paragraph, for drugs with long $t_{1/2}$, especially if longer than 24 hours (e.g., about 70 hours for teicoplanin, 40 hours for digoxin, 96 hours for phenobarbital), the initial administra-

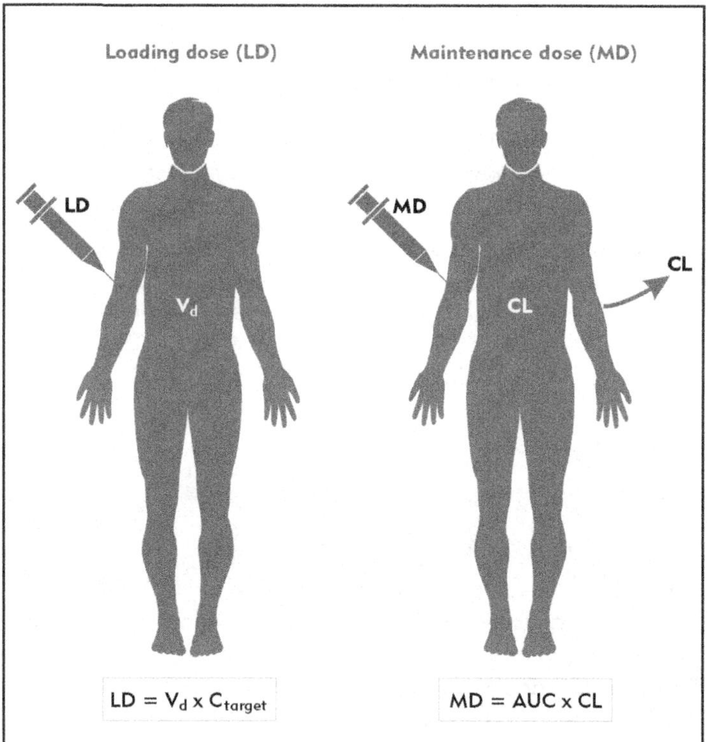

Figure 14. Loading dose and maintenance dose.

tion of an LD allows the rapid achievement of concentrations similar to the C_{ss}, which otherwise would take several days from starting therapy.
In such circumstances, once that the LD has been administered at the beginning of therapy, in the following days the treatment will be continued with an MD which should substantially correspond to the amount of drug necessary for the replacement of the moiety that has been eliminated by the excretory organs during the dosing interval. Therefore, it follows that the MD, differently from the LD, depends only on the CL of the drug.
Because it represents the amount of drug that must be administered in order to replace the moiety that was removed, the following formula is used for its calculation (Figure 14):

$$MD = AUC \times CL$$

1.8.1 | Clinical Meaning of LD and MD

The clinical meaning of the LD and the MD in everyday practice depends essentially on the intrinsic pharmacokinetic characteristics of each drug and on the patient's therapeutic needs, related to his/her clinical situation. Accordingly, the initial administration of an LD is mandatory whenever a rapid therapeutic response to drugs with long $t_{1/2}$ is needed.
This procedure may become a strong recommendation in relation to the type of therapy: for example, the treatment of bacterial infections with teicoplanin always requires an LD because this approach allows either a more rapid therapeutic response or a better microbiological eradication with prevention of the spread of resistance due to drug underexposure.
However, for some drugs with long $t_{1/2}$, the use of the LD is recommended only in certain particular circumstances. This is the case for some drugs with low therapeutic index, or drugs with narrow therapeutic range (i.e., having little difference between the toxic and the therapeutic doses). For example, this is the case of the therapeutic use of digoxin for the treatment of heart failure in intensive care in which the so-called rapid

digitalization is adopted. Similar considerations can be made also with regard to the treatment of status epilepticus with phenobarbital or diazepam.
Indeed, for low therapeutic index drugs having long $t_{1/2}$, as precautionary measure, application of the LD is mainly restricted to the hospital settings in which it is easier to monitor the patient in relation to the possible risk of major adverse reactions related to excessively high drug concentrations.

2 PHARMACOKINETICS AND POLYTHERAPY

Theoretically, the pharmacokinetic drug-drug interactions during polytherapy may concern each of the four phases of pharmacokinetics (absorption, distribution, metabolism, and excretion). In practice, as we shall see, the majority of these events occur during the phases of absorption or of metabolism. This is because many drugs that need biotransformation to be eliminated share the enzyme systems responsible for their metabolism. In fact, these systems are devoted to modify some structural components of the drug, such as COOH, NH_2 groups, etc., and not the drug as a whole. The clinical-pharmacological result of this is that many drugs can be substrates of the same enzyme system, irrespective of having different structural characteristics and different therapeutic uses.

To better understand the pathophysiological basis of pharmacokinetic drug-drug interactions, it is important to consider the functioning of the main physiological systems that regulate these processes, namely, the cytochrome enzymes (CYP) P450 and the transmembrane P170 glycoprotein (Pgp).

2.1 Cytochrome P450 (CYP)

The cytochrome P450 (CYP) enzyme system is the major responsible for the oxidative metabolism of drugs in the liver. It represents the most significant route for the elimination of drugs from the body, and the main cause of pharmacokinetic drug-drug interactions during polytherapy. In humans, several families of enzymes are expressed, the so-called isoforms. Among these, the most relevant from a clinical-pharmacological point of view

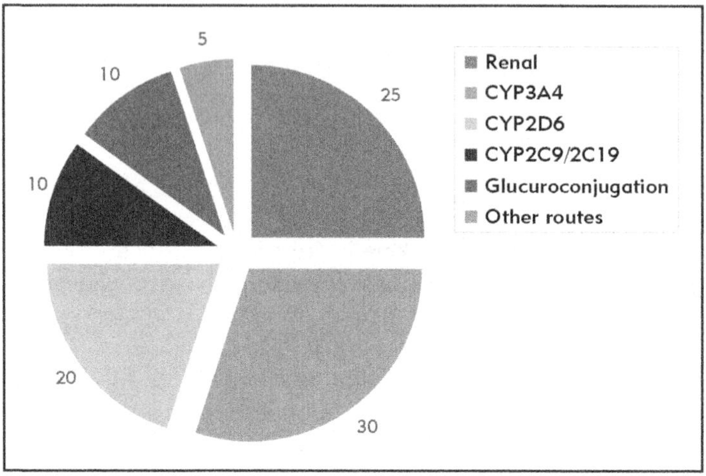

Figure 15. Incidence (%) of the main routes of elimination of drugs.

are the CYP3A4, the CYP2D6, the CYP2C19, the CYP2C9, the CYP1A2, and to a lesser extent, the CYP2E1 (Figure 15).
A common feature to all of the drugs that are metabolized by CYP450 (substrates) is their high lipophilicity.
Pharmacokinetic interactions of considerable clinical relevance may occur whenever the activity of the various CYP450 isoforms is changed as a result of substances that reduce or increase the efficiency of the metabolizing system. These substances are defined, respectively, as enzymatic **inhibitors** and **inducers**. Generally speaking, the **enzymatic inhibitors** are substances capable of binding to the enzyme, often irreversibly, thus blocking its activity. Conversely, the **enzymatic inducers** are substances that increase the amount of translation of genetic information coding for the production of these enzymes. It follows therefore that, in presence of an enzymatic inhibitor, the major pharmacokinetic effect which occurs with regard to a drug that is a CYP450 substrate is the decrease of its CL and consequently an increase of its exposure (AUC). Therefore, being AUC = dose/CL, in the absence of dose reduction, this leads to drug accumulation, thus increasing the potential risk of toxicity (Figure 16).

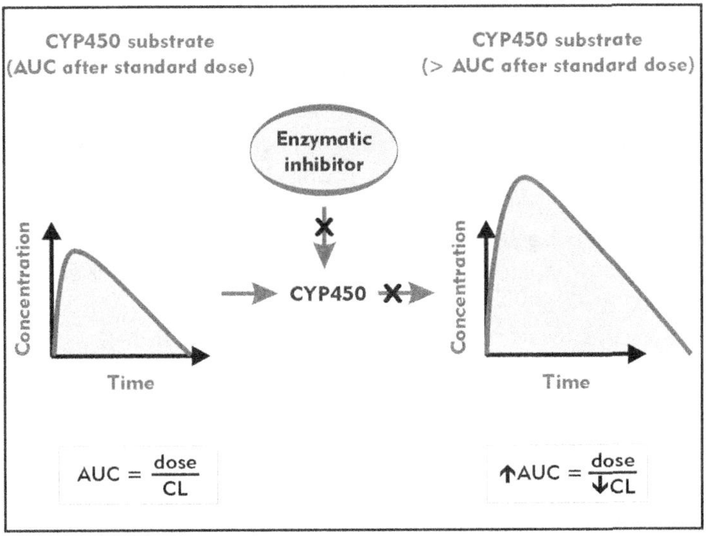

Figure 16. Pharmacokinetic interaction due to inhibition of CYP450.

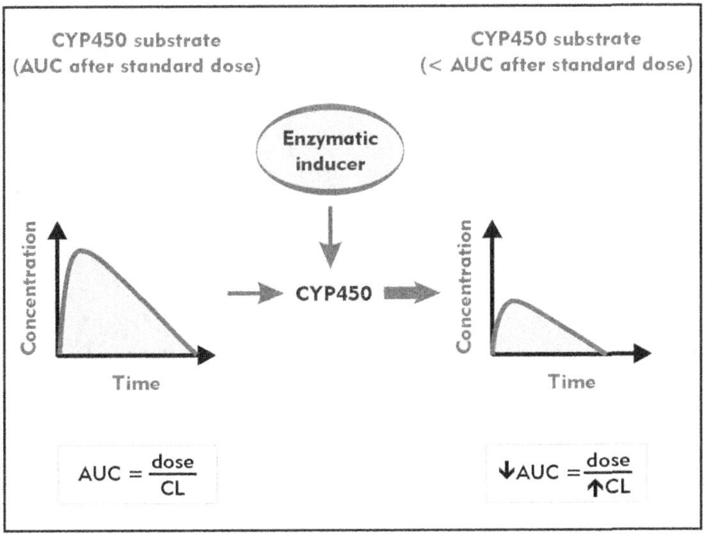

Figure 17. Pharmacokinetic interaction due to induction of CYP450.

On the contrary, in the presence of an enzymatic inducer, the main pharmacokinetic effect that occurs with regard to a medication which is a CYP450 substrate is an increase in its CL and consequently a reduction of its exposure (AUC). Therefore, in the absence of a dosage increase, this effect causes a risk of treatment failure due to underexposure (Figure 17).
It is noteworthy that sometimes the magnitude of the enzymatic inhibition can be so powerful to determine, for example, an increase in drug exposure (AUC) of the drug substrate used at standard dose of even 4-6 folds.
In theory this would require a corresponding dose reduction (by 4-6 folds compared to standard dose) of the drug substrate, but in some cases it is preferred simply to contraindicate the combination of the two drugs in order to prevent any toxicity risk. On the other hand, after a powerful effect of enzymatic induction it may happen that drug exposure at the standard dose of the substrate is reduced by more than 70-80% with the consequent need to increase the dose of 4-5 folds.
Here are reported some examples of possible clinically relevant pharmacokinetic interactions in relation to the different isoforms of CYP450 to which it is necessary to pay attention in case of polytherapy.

2.1.1 | CYP3A4

The CYP3A4 is the primary mechanism of oxidative-reductive biotransformation. Many drugs in various therapeutic classes, such as benzodiazepines, calcium channel blockers and immunosuppressive drugs, are substrates of CYP3A4 and, therefore, it is not surprising that in patients on polytherapy regimens, pharmacokinetic interactions involving this isoform can frequently occur. The following are the main substrates of CYP3A4, as well as the main enzymatic inhibitors and inducers, which can cause an increase or decrease, respectively, in exposure of the substrates, and thus an enhancement or a reduction in their effect (Figure 18).
However, it must be highlighted that not all the drugs belonging to the same therapeutic class have the same behavior with

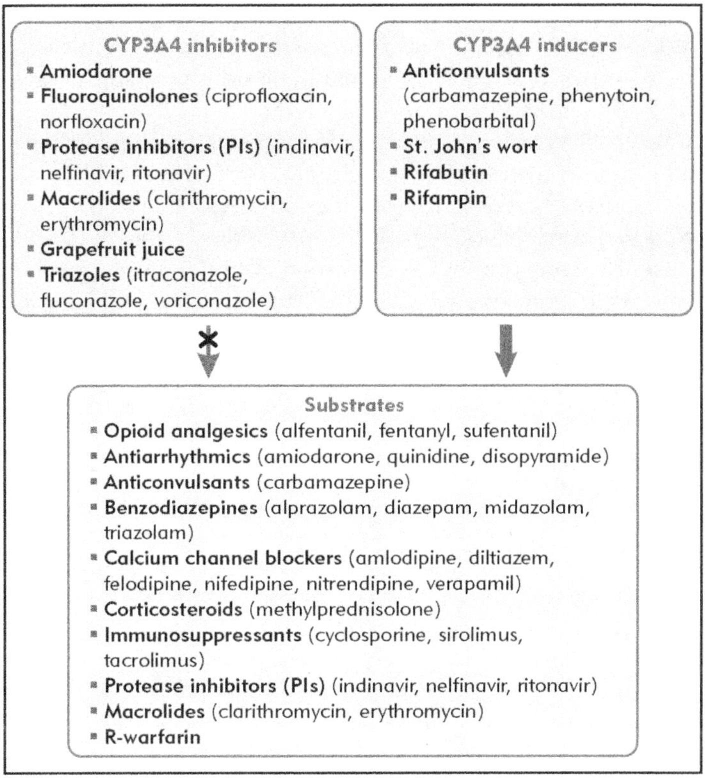

Figure 18. Pharmacokinetic interactions of CYP3A4.

Drug	Elimination route
Atorvastatin	**CYP3A4**
Cerivastatin	**CYP3A4**; CYP2C8
Fluvastatin	CYP2C9
Lovastatin	**CYP3A4**
Pravastatin	Sulfation
Rosuvastatin	Fecal, renal
Simvastatin	**CYP3A4**

Table VI. Statins and elimination route.

regard to CYP3A4, either as substrates or as inducers or as inhibitors, but this depends on their physicochemical characteristics. As an example, consider that not all statins are substrates of CYP3A4 (Table VI).

This means, for example, that whereas the concomitant intake of atorvastatin, lovastatin or simvastatin with CYP3A4 inhibitors may cause an increased risk of rhabdomyolysis due to overexposure to these inhibitors of cholesterol synthesis, this does not represent a contraindication for other statins, such as rosuvastatin, which are not substrates of this isoenzyme. Similarly, some fluoroquinolones act as inhibitors of CYP3A4 (e.g., ciprofloxacin), but others do not (e.g., levofloxacin, moxifloxacin). Furthermore, this enzymatic system has two relevant characteristics from the clinical point of view. The first is the fact that this isoform is largely expressed, not only in the liver, but also in the gut wall.

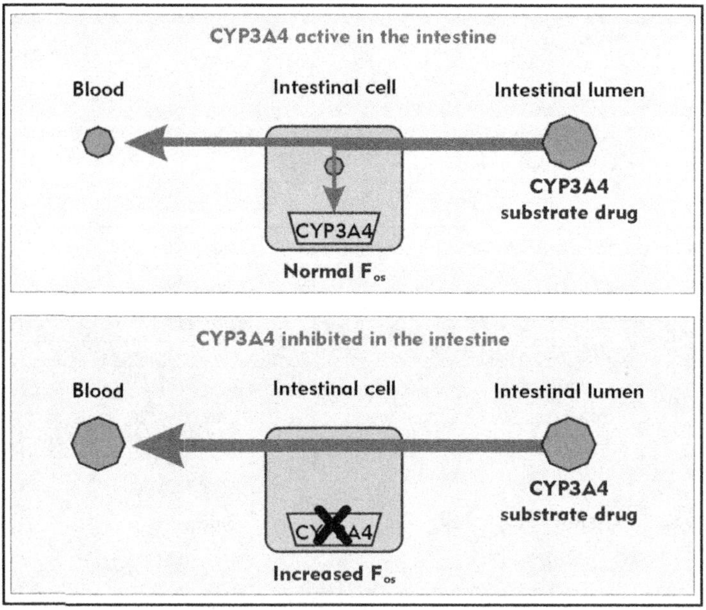

Figure 19. F_{os} in the presence of a CYP3A4 inhibitor.

This phenomenon can explain why the F_{os} of some drugs that are CYP3A4 substrates may significantly change as a result of the concomitant administration of substances that are able to modify CYP3A4 activity. In the presence of an inhibitor of CYP3A4, there will be an increase in F_{os} (Figure 19), while in the presence of an inducer there will be a decrease in F_{os} (Figure 20).

The second aspect that is important to highlight is that, in addition to drugs *sensu strictu*, there are other substances that may alter the activity profile of CYP3A4. Among these, we must surely remember grapefruit juice and St. John's wort.

Grapefruit juice acts as an inhibitor of CYP3A4, because it contains a series of coumarin derivatives (dihydroxybergamottin) and bioflavonoids (naringin, naringenin, quercetin) that block its activity.

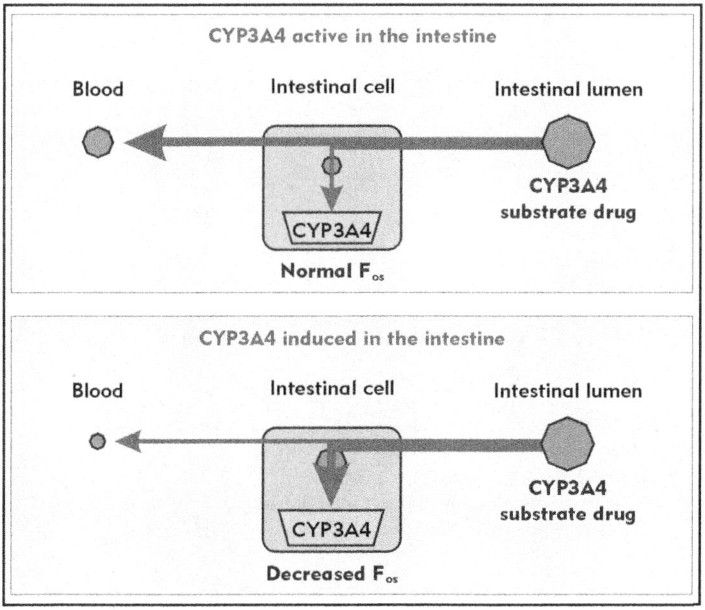

Figure 20. F_{os} in the presence of a CYP3A4 inducer.

It is interesting to point out that long-term consumption can cause greater inhibitory effects—in terms of intensity and duration—than occasional consumption. From these considerations it therefore seems clear that oral intake of drugs that are substrates of CYP3A4 with grapefruit juice may be harmful, as this may result in a significant increase in their F_{os} and AUC and, consequently, of adverse effects due to overexposure. For example, it has been shown that oral assumption of a calcium channel blocker with a glass of grapefruit juice may result in a significant increase of drug exposure (AUC), with more potent hypotensive effect as pharmacodynamic consequence.
Conversely, *Hypericum perforatum* (or St. John's wort)—a herbaceous plant widespread in Europe whose extract, taken orally, is sometimes used for its antiviral and antidepressant properties—is an inducer of CYP3A4. Therefore, during treatment with hypericum, the oral intake of drugs that are substrates of CYP3A4 may result in therapeutic failure, as a consequence of a significant decrease in F_{os} and AUC.

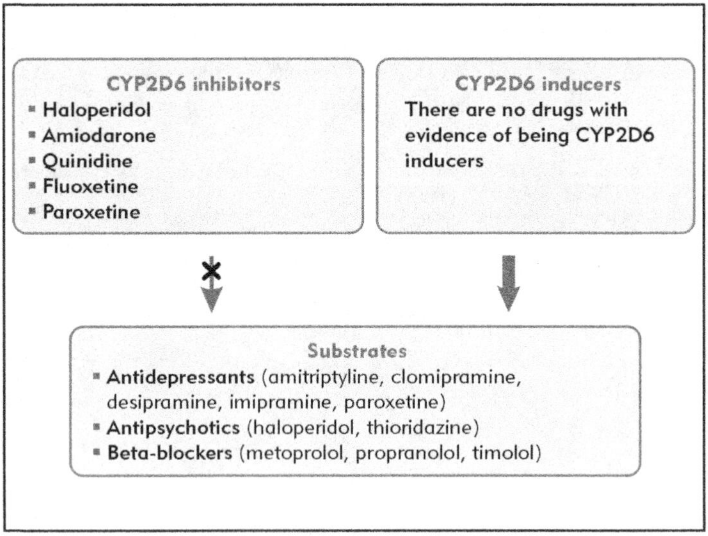

Figure 21. Pharmacokinetic interactions of CYP2D6.

2.1.2 | CYP2D6

CYP2D6 represents about 1.5% of the CYP isoforms in the human liver and is implicated in the metabolism of some beta-blockers, antidepressants and antipsychotics. Its activity can be inhibited by the co-administration of certain antidepressants (fluoxetine, paroxetine) or antiarrhythmics (amiodarone, quinidine). Figure 21 shows the main substrates, inhibitors and inducers of CYP2D6, that may be involved in pharmacokinetic interactions of clinical significance.

2.1.3 | CYP2C19

CYP2C19 is the major route of metabolism of proton pump inhibitors (Figure 22).

A peculiar aspect of this isoform that may have clinical relevance is the fact that it is characterized by a genetic polymorphism, that is a genetically predetermined variation of its expression:

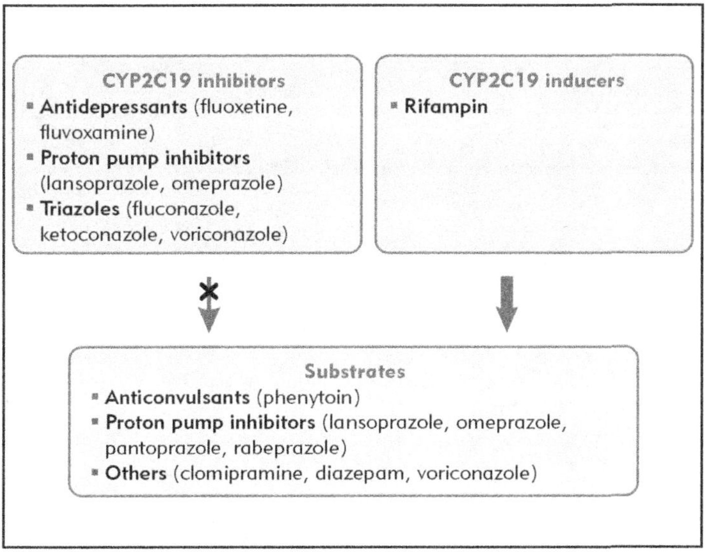

Figure 22. Pharmacokinetic interactions of CYP2C19.

while most of the population have a suitable amount of enzyme (extensive metabolizers), about 2% of the Caucasian population and 20% of the Asian one are almost completely deficient of this enzyme (poor metabolizers).
This may explain why in poor metabolizers of CYP2C19, standard doses of drugs that are substrate of this enzyme may cause an increased exposure (AUC), and therefore a potential risk of toxicity, even when these drugs are used in the absence of concomitant intake of enzymatic inhibitors.

2.1.4 | CYP2C9

CYP2C9 is generally about one-third of the total content of CYPs in the liver and is implicated in the metabolism of more than 100 drugs, including anticoagulants, sulfonylureas, and some anti-inflammatory drugs (NSAIDs) (Figure 23).

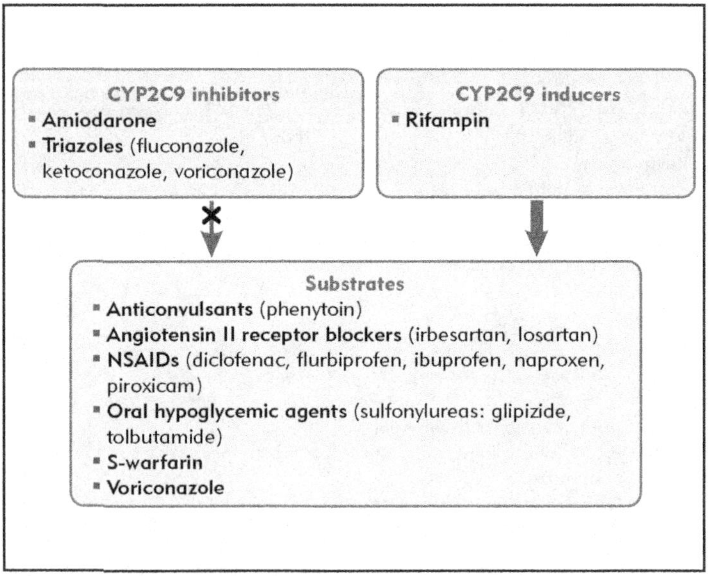

Figure 23. Pharmacokinetic interactions of CYP2C9.

2.1.5 | CYP1A2

CYP1A2 accounts for approximately 10-15% of the activity of CYP450 in the liver and, among others, is responsible for the metabolism of theophylline and of the right- (R-) enantiomer of warfarin. Its activity is inhibited by ciprofloxacin and fluoxetine and conversely is induced by carbamazepine and rifampicin (Figure 24).

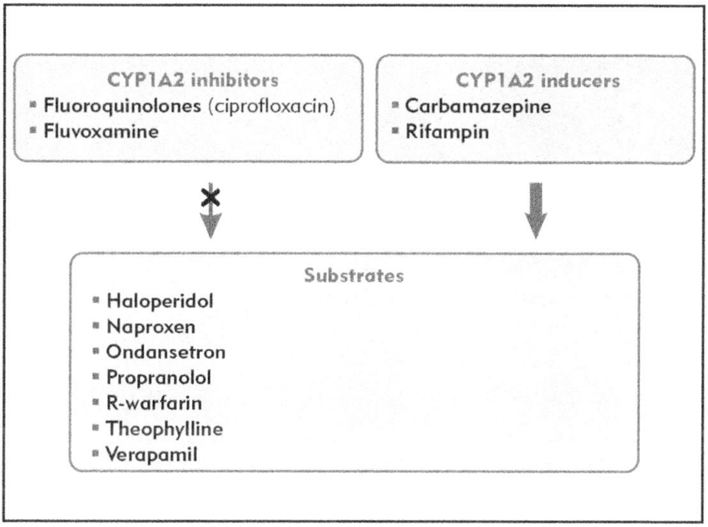

Figure 24. Pharmacokinetic interactions of CYP1A2.

2.2 P170 Glycoprotein (Pgp)

The P170 glycoprotein (Pgp) is a transmembrane protein normally present in many human cells that acts as a protective and detoxifying extrusive pump against many xenobiotics. Since it is widely present in the intestine, in the excretory organs (liver, kidney) and in the blood-brain barrier, it follows that many drugs, being xenobiotics, may be its substrates (Table VII).

Analgesics	• Morphine
Antibiotics	• Erythromycin, rifampin
Antidepressants	• Paroxetine, venlafaxine
Antiepileptics	• Carbamazepine, lamotrigine, phenobarbital, phenytoin
Antineoplastics	• Vinca alkaloids: vinblastine, vincristine • Taxanes: docetaxel, paclitaxel • Anthracyclines: doxorubicin, daunorubicin, epirubicin, idarubicin • Epipodophyllotoxins: etoposide, teniposide • Others: actinomycin, irinotecan, methotrexate, mitomycin, tamoxifen, topotecan
Antivirals	• Protease inhibitors
Calcium blockers	• Verapamil
Cardiac glycosides	• Digoxin
Immunosuppressors	• Cyclosporin A, tacrolimus
Protom pump inhibitors	• Lansoprazole, omeprazole, pantoprazole

Table VII. Examples of drugs that are substrates of Pgp.

It was recently demonstrated that the activity of Pgp is modulable and it has therefore been hypothesized that many pharmacokinetic interactions that occur during polytherapy may be consequent to alterations in the Pgp activity. In particular, it has

Antiarrhythmics	• Amiodarone, quinidine, verapamil
Antibiotics	• Clarithromycin, erythromycin
Antidepressants	• Paroxetine, sertraline
Antineoplastics	• Doxorubicin, vinblastine
Proton pump inhibitors	• Esomeprazole, lansoprazole, omeprazole, pantoprazole
Others	• Cyclosporin A

Table VIII. Examples of drugs that are inhibitors of Pgp.

been shown that some drugs of various therapeutic classes are able to inhibit its activity (Table VIII).
The consequences of the co-administration of a drug that acts as a Pgp inhibitor toward a drug that is a substrate of Pgp have an impact at two levels: on the one hand, inhibition of intestinal Pgp causes an increase in oral bioavailability (> F_{os}) (Figure 25), and on the other hand, inhibition of Pgp at the level of the excretory organs causes reduced elimination (< CL) (Figure 26).
Thus, exposure to the drug substrate can be significantly increased (> AUC). Indeed, currently, only some of these potential interactions have been clearly recognized as clinically relevant, such in the case of the co-administration of amiodarone or some macrolides with digoxin (with decreased CL of digoxin and consequent risk of digitalis intoxication).

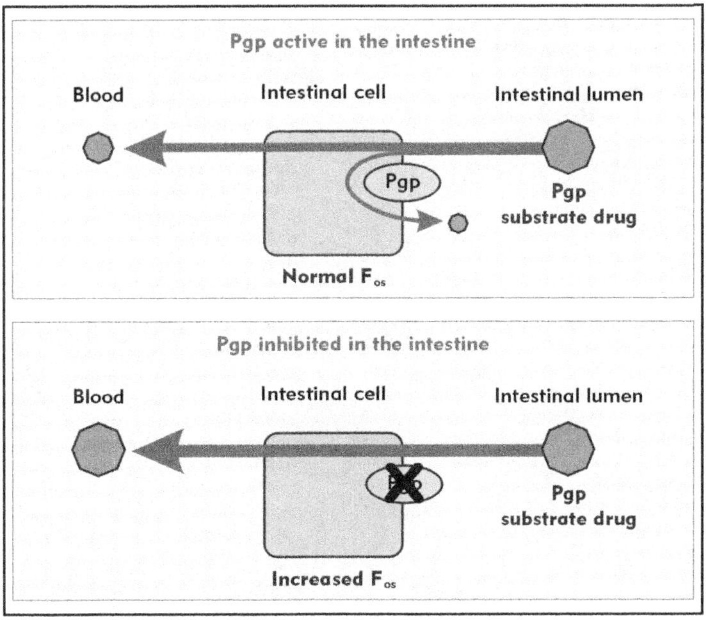

Figure 25. Pgp in the intestine.

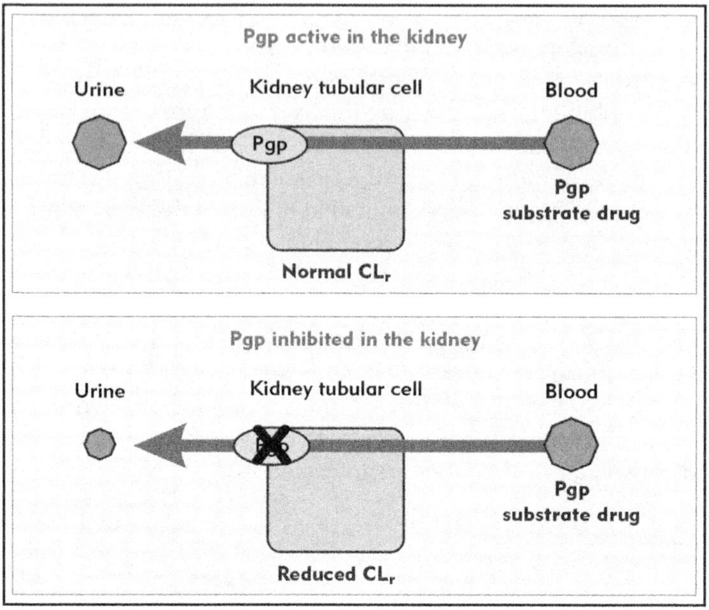

Figure 26. Pgp in the kidney.

3 PHARMACOKINETICS AND DOSING REGIMEN

Pharmacokinetic studies that are performed in the initial phase of clinical trials of a drug are usually carried out in healthy volunteers. These studies are mainly aimed at finding out the "fate" of the drug in the body, in order to identify the best dose to achieve the desired therapeutic effect.
In other words, these studies help to define the dosing regimen of a drug, i.e., which amount of dose should be administered and how often it should be given. This is based on the evaluation of the profile of plasma concentrations over time in relation to increasing doses of the drug (dose finding studies) with the aim of identifying the type of kinetics and the routes of elimination.
A detailed analysis of these concepts is beyond the purpose of this publication. However, it should not be overlooked that the pharmacokinetic studies carried out for regulatory purposes are usually performed in healthy volunteers, who of course, by definition, are not patients.
This obvious consideration should force to think over the fact that whenever a patient has pathophysiological conditions which may alter the pharmacokinetic behavior of the drugs in the body, dosage adjustments will be needed in order to always guarantee drug concentrations similar to those that have been defined as therapeutically effective in *ad hoc* studies.

4 PHARMACOKINETICS AND PATIENT PATHOPHYSIOLOGY

In a perhaps simplistic, but yet extremely effective, way it is possible to represent the pharmacokinetics of a drug in the body with a metaphorical example.
In fact, the maintenance of therapeutically effective concentrations of the drug at the site of action (C_{ss}), which is a prerequisite for appropriate therapy, can be imagined as the result of the balance between inputs and outputs.
The inputs are represented by the amount of the drug that is administered (the dose), whereas the outputs by the amount of drug that is eliminated (CL).
The C_{ss} of a drug becomes stable when inputs and outputs are equal and, as aforementioned, this happens more or less after a period of time of 4-5 times its $t_{1/2}$ from starting therapy.
Remember that the C_{ss} is really steady only if the drug has been administered by continuous intravenous infusion.
In fact, in such circumstances, the amount of drug eliminated through the excretory organs is replaced second by second via continuous administration of the drug according to the formula:

$$IR\ (\mu g/min) = C_{ss}\ (\mu g/ml) \times CL\ (ml/min)$$

A scheme that can help to understand this formula is to imagine the human body as a container in which the C_{ss} of the drug is the result of the perfect balance between the administered amount (IR) and the eliminated one (CL) (Figure 27).
From this scheme it appears that whenever the stationary conditions will change, due to variation of the dosage (IR) or of the CL or of both, as a consequence the C_{ss} will be alterated and will have to be achieved again.

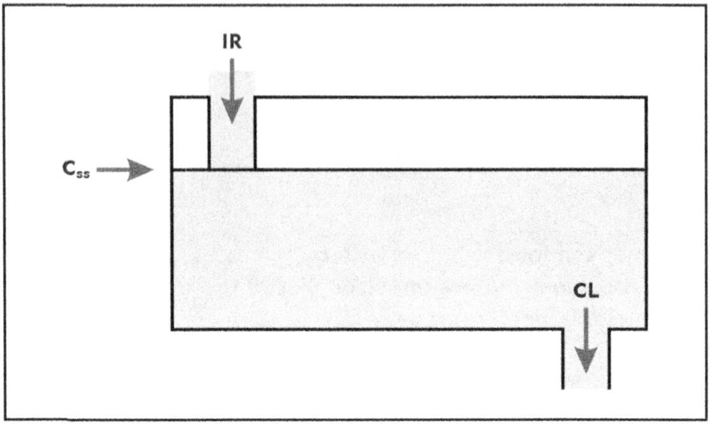

Figure 27. Balance between the administered (IR) and the eliminated (CL) moiety of the drug.

Similarly, if a therapy is carried out intermittently and not continuously, the plasma exposure to the drug, rather than remaining perfectly constant over time, fluctuates repeatedly between a minimum ($C_{ss\ min}$) and a maximum ($C_{ss\ max}$) in relation to the frequency of administration. In this case we can represent the exposure in terms of AUC instead of C_{ss}, as follows:

$$MD\ (\mu g) = AUC\ (\mu g/ml \times min) \times CL\ (ml/min)$$

From this formula the AUC may be extrapolated:

$$AUC = \frac{MD}{CL}$$

It follows therefore that, if the CL of a drug varies due to a change in the functionality of the excretory organs responsible for its elimination, if the dose that is administered to the patient is maintained unchanged, a significant change in the AUC, namely in the daily exposure to the drug, will occur.
In particular, if the CL decreases, drug exposure will be larger, and this will result in an increased risk of toxicity (Figure 28).

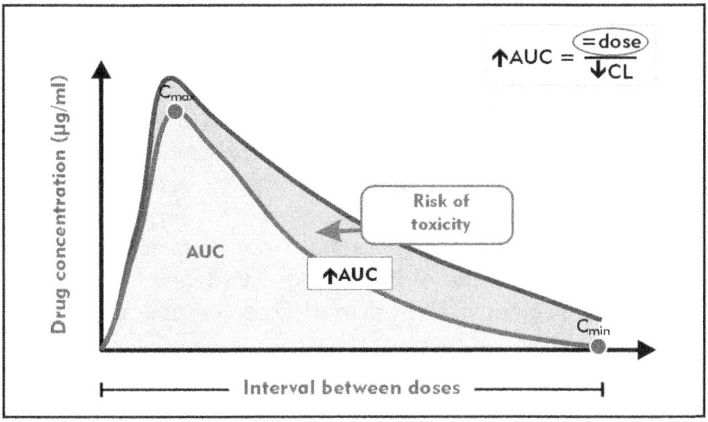

Figure 28. Plasma drug exposure and descreased clearance: risk of toxicity.

Conversely, if the CL increases, drug exposure will be lower, and this will lead to the risk of potential treatment failure (Figure 29). Here below are described those pathophysiological conditions which may alter the pharmacokinetic profile of a drug.

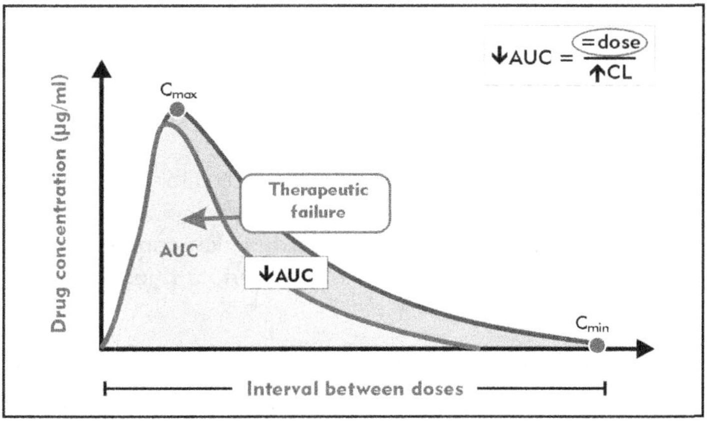

Figure 29. Plasma drug exposure and increased clearance: risk of treatment failure.

4.1 Age

Age significantly affects the pharmacokinetic behavior of many drugs. The pharmacokinetic changes that occur with age are the result of some major physiological changes: on the one hand, changes in the composition of body tissues and of water content, and on the other hand, changes in the function of the excretory organs. Such considerations are helpful to explain why the pharmacokinetic studies needed to define the dosing regimen of a given drug must be performed in subpopulations of individuals stratified by age.
However, it was recently shown that the distinction based on four different age groups—newborns, pediatrics, adults and elderly—which was proposed until some time ago, turned out to be insufficient to appropriately describe the dosage adjustments needed to ensure adequate drug exposure in all of the patients. In fact, in relation to the significant increase in life expectancy, it was shown that within the range of the elderly population, the pharmacokinetics of a given drug can vary considerably in individuals older than 80 years compared to those aged 65 years. Therefore, based on the current scientific evidence, it is believed that from a pharmacokinetic point of view it is better to consider, at least five age groups: newborns, pediatrics, adults, elderly, and very elderly.

4.1.1 | Newborns and Pediatrics vs. Adults

The selection of an appropriate dose of medication in the neonatal period must reflect the process of physiological development that has not yet been completed, which can obviously have a number of consequences on the various phases of the pharmacokinetics (Table IX).

Absorption

With regard to absorption, it is considered that gastric pH is almost neutral at birth and decreases slowly to reach values similar to that of the adults by around 2 years of age.

Physiological factor	Neonatal period	Childhood	Altered pharmacokinetic phase
Gastric pH	Neutral	Acid	Absorption
Gastric emptying time	Prolonged	Normal after 6-8 months	Absorption
Intestinal motility	Reduced	Increased	Absorption
Muscle blood flow	Reduced and unpredictable	Increased	Absorption
Intestinal CYP3A4	Reduced	Normal	Absorption
Total body water	80-90%	60% after 1 year	Distribution
Extracellular water	45%	25%	Distribution
Drug-protein binding	Reduced	Normal	Distribution
Blood-brain barrier	Immature	Normal only after 4-6 years	Distribution
Phase I reactions	Reduced	Normal after 3 months	Metabolism
Phase II reactions	Reduced	Normal after 3 months	Metabolism
Hepatic blood flow	Reduced	Increased	Metabolism
Renal blood flow	Reduced	Increased	Elimination
Renal glomerular filtration	Reduced	Normal after 6 months	Elimination
Renal tubular secretion	Reduced	Normal after 6-12 months	Elimination

Table IX. Physiological factors that influence pharmacokinetics in the neonatal period and early childhood.

CYP3A4 = P450 isoform 3A4 of cytochrome P450

It follows that in the first weeks of life the absorption of acid-labile drugs (e.g., erythromycin) will be more efficient, whereas, conversely, that of drugs which are weak acids (e.g., phenobarbital and phenytoin) will be reduced. The gastric emptying

time is prolonged in the first months of life and reaches values similar to those of the adults only at around 6-8 months of age. Therefore, in this period the absorption of certain drugs may be delayed (e.g., paracetamol), and therefore a longer latency in the onset of their therapeutic effect may be observed. The intestinal transit is prolonged as a result of decreased intestinal motility in the first months of life, but on the contrary tends to be increased in early childhood, and this may lead to incomplete absorption. The absorption after intramuscular administration is erratic in infants, as the muscle blood flow is extremely variable. Therefore, administration of drugs by this route (e.g., benzodiazepine) should be avoided during this period.
The activity of CYP3A4 in the gut wall is reduced in the first 2 weeks of life. It follows therefore that the F_{os} of some drugs metabolized by this enzyme (e.g., midazolam) can be increased as a result of a reduced first-pass effect.

Distribution

Regarding the distribution of drugs, it should be taken into consideration that in the neonatal period the total body water is 80-90% of body weight, with a progressive decrease occurring with age, approaching 55-60% in adults. Moreover, whereas in the neonatal period the amount of extracellular water is approximately 45% of body weight, it drops to 20% in adulthood. Consequently, in the neonatal period many hydrophilic drugs, such as beta-lactam and aminoglycoside antibiotics, have considerably larger V_d in comparison with those observed in childhood or adulthood, and thus the initial LD of these drugs should be larger.
It should also be noted that the plasma protein binding is reduced in the neonatal period; and, therefore, drugs that are normally more than 90% bound (e.g., many anti-inflammatory drugs), may present a larger free moiety that is biologically active. Finally, the blood-brain barrier is immature until about 6 years of life. Therefore hydrophilic drugs may cross the barrier with relative ease in this period of life, differently from what occurs in adulthood when they may diffuse into the central

nervous system only in situations of altered permeability (e.g., meningitis).
This may allow to explain, for example, the greater frequency of adverse events of the central nervous system (e.g., irritability, insomnia, abnormal behavior) that may be encountered during the first years of life following the administration of high doses of beta-lactam antibiotics.

Metabolism

Regarding metabolic activity, it should be taken into consideration that both phase I and phase II enzymes are often immature at birth (Figure 30).
In particular, the acetylation processes reach full activity about 20 days after birth, those of conjugation with glucuronic acid and many of those mediated by CYP450 isoforms after about 2-3 months, and those of conjugation with aminoacids after about 3 months.
Overall, it is believed that the complete maturation of liver enzymes is reached after about 1 year of age. It appears, therefore, that in this period of life it may be necessary to reduce the doses of certain drugs compared to older ages, or it may

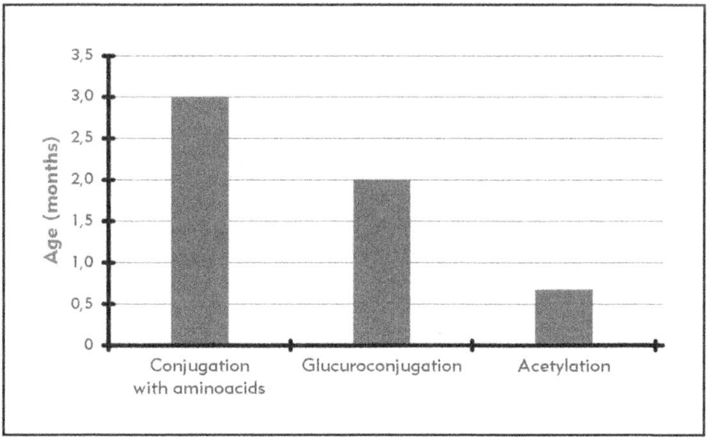

Figure 30. Postnatal development of hepatic functions.

be even necessary to avoid their use. As an example, recall the neonatal chloramphenicol toxicity ("gray syndrome") that occurs due to the accumulation of the drug caused by a deficiency of glucuronosyl transferase activities. In general, it is believed that the period of most rapid hepatic CL coincides with school age and adolescence, and that then a progressive decrease with age may occur.

Elimination

Finally, as regards elimination, it should be taken into consideration that while the glomerular filtration is completed by 1 month of age, mainly due to the progressive increase in renal blood flow during the first weeks of life, conversely active tubular secretion is not efficient until between the 6th and the 12th month of life (Figure 31).

It follows, therefore, that in the neonatal period the CL_r of drugs can be lower than at later ages.

Regarding the assessment of the extent of glomerular filtration rate on the basis of serum creatinine, the Schwartz formula, which takes into account these differences, is the one usually used to estimate creatinine clearance in children:

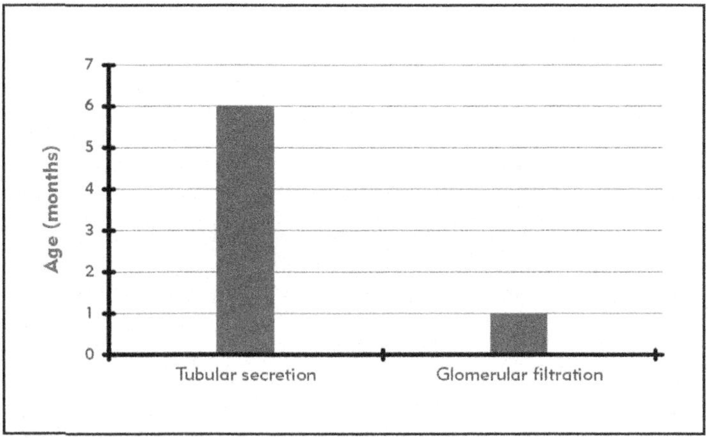

Figure 31. Postnatal development of renal function.

$$CL_{cr} = \frac{\text{Height (cm)} \times K}{S_{cr}}$$

where:

- K is a constant equal to:
  - 0.4 if premature
  - 0.45 if born at term < 1 year
  - 0.5 if 1-2 years old
  - 0.55 if 2-12 years old
- CL_{cr} = creatinine clearance
- S_{cr} = serum creatinine

In children older than 12 years, the Cockcroft and Gault formula can be applied (see below).

4.1.2 | Elderly

Elderly patients may present some physiological changes due to aging processes, which may affect the pharmacokinetic behavior of many drugs (Table X).

Physiological change vs. adults	Pharmacokinetic consequence
Slow gastric emptying	> t_{max}
< intestinal CYP3A4 activity	> F_{os} of drugs that are substrate of CYP3A4
< total body water	> concentration of hydrophilic drugs
> body fat	> V_d and $t_{1/2}$ for lipophilic drugs
< hepatic blood flow	< CL for drugs with "high hepatic extraction"
< phase I enzymes activity	< CL and > $t_{1/2}$ for lipophilic drugs metabolized by CYP450
≈ phase II enzymes activity	≈ CL and ≈ $t_{1/2}$ for lipophilic drugs metabolized by conjugation processes
< glomerular filtration	< CL and > $t_{1/2}$ for hydrophilic drugs

Table X. Physiological changes in the elderly compared to adults, and their pharmacokinetic consequences.

Absorption

In elderly patients gastric emptying is slowed down and intestinal peristalsis is reduced.

These effects can cause a prolongation of time to reach the maximum concentration (t_{max}) of some drugs after oral administration with consequent increase in the latency of onset of the therapeutic effect.

Additionally, the first-pass effect is reduced due to the decreased activity of CYP3A4 in the intestinal wall. Consequently, drugs that are substrates of CYP3A4 present an increased F_{os}. Of note, the F_{os} of some antihypertensive drugs (such as labetalol, propranolol, and verapamil) was shown to be almost doubled in the elderly compared to that observed in the adults.

Distribution

The composition of body tissues changes consistently with age (Figure 32).

Of note, in people aged over 65 years lean body mass and water content (50% of body weight) are significantly decreased,

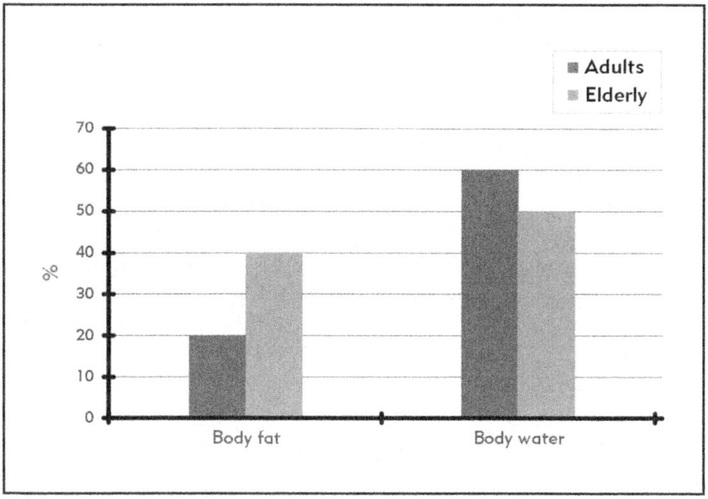

Figure 32. Change in composition of body tissues with age.

whereas adipose tissue increases, especially in females (30% in males and 40% in females). The main pharmacokinetic consequences of these events are the decrease in V_d for hydrophilic drugs with consequent increase in their plasma concentration and, conversely, the increase in V_d for lipophilic drugs with consequent prolongation of their $t_{1/2}$.

Metabolism

Aging causes a reduction of hepatic blood flow by about 40% compared to adulthood.

Consequently, in elderly patients the CL of drugs with high liver extraction rate is significantly reduced. Additionally, the enzymatic processes responsible for the biotransformation of drugs may undergo a different degree of impairment with aging. It has been estimated that the activity of phase I enzymes is significantly reduced in the elderly. As a consequence, it was shown that the $t_{1/2}$ of many drugs that are substrates of CYP450 undergoes an average increase of about 80% compared to that observed in 20-30-year-old adults. By contrast, the activity of phase II enzymes (or synthetic enzymes) is only slightly modified by aging. Therefore, the $t_{1/2}$ of drugs eliminated by conjugation processes is similar to that found in the adult population.

Elimination

Glomerular filtration is consistently reduced with age. Several case studies show that the average decrease of glomerular filtration rate observed in the elderly ranges between 13% and 68%. This appears to be the result of the progressive glomerulosclerosis which, on average, affects 15-20% of the glomeruli in people older than 65-70 years. It follows, therefore, that the $t_{1/2}$ of drugs that are renally eliminated is significantly extended in the elderly, by an average of 30-50% compared to adults.

Estimation of glomerular filtration rate by means of the Cockcroft and Gault formula becomes particularly helpful for appropriate management of the dosage of drugs eliminated by the

kidney in the treatment of elderly patients, especially when the values of serum creatinine (S_{cr}) are within the normal ranges from the clinical point of view.
The Cockcroft and Gault formula is expressed as follows:

- **males**

$$CL_{cr} = \frac{140 - age}{72 \times S_{cr}} \times weight$$

- **females**

$$CL_{cr} = males \times 0.85$$

This aspect of delayed renal elimination of drugs acquires additional importance in the very-elderly population, namely people aged over 85 years, since it is likely that the process of glomerulosclerosis becomes even more relevant, thus causing a further significant impairment of glomerular filtration rate.
In conclusion, it is clear from the foregoing that in the elderly population there is a series of physiological changes that lead to an increase of the residence time of the drugs in the body. In other words, in the elderly drugs exhibit often $t_{1/2}$ much longer than observed in the young, and this means that careful attention should be paid to the posology, by using the "right" dose, which in many cases will be significantly lower than that used in the adult population. Obviously, this approach is fundamental in preventing the risk of adverse events, whose incidence in the elderly population is frequently increased, according to many published studies. Although some adverse reactions are certainly due to pharmacodynamic aspects (e.g., higher receptor sensitivity), however a significant proportion of these is certainly related to the drug overexposure, in terms of AUC, which may be the consequence of the fact that no dosage adjustment in relation to the changed pathophysiological conditions was taken into account.

Example

To explain how age may affect the choice of the correct dose of medication, we describe the case of two persons who have the same physiological characteristics (male, weight 72 kg, S_{cr} = 1 mg/dl), but who differ in age (18 vs. 75 years):

- 1° subject: male, 18 years old, weight 72 kg, S_{cr} = 1 mg/dl
- 2° subject: male, 75 years old, weight 72 kg, S_{cr} = 1 mg/dl

By substituting the values of weight and S_{cr} in the Cockcroft and Gault formula, we note that the only factor that influences a difference in the CL_{cr} estimates of these two patients is represented by age:

$$\mathbf{CL_{cr} = \frac{(140 - age) \times 72}{72 \times 1}}$$

By simplifying the formula, we have:

$$\mathbf{CL_{cr} = 140 - age}$$

Therefore, in the young aged 18:

$$\mathbf{CL_{cr} = 140 - 18 = 122\ ml/min}$$

whereas in the elderly aged 75:

$$\mathbf{CL_{cr} = 140 - 75 = 65\ ml/min}$$

Since the daily exposure to a drug (AUC) is the result of the administered dose and of the total body CL (AUC = dose/CL) and since for drugs eliminated by the kidney there is a linear relationship between the drug CL and the CL_{cr}, it follows that the elderly patient, by having in this case a CL_{cr} halved compared to that of the younger (65 vs. 122 ml/min) will have a halved drug CL_r, so that he/she has to receive half dose (AUC dose = 0.5/0.5 CL) in order to have the same drug exposure of the younger patient (AUC = dose/CL) and to avoid an increased risk of toxicity.

4.2 Renal Failure

Many drugs have exclusive or predominant renal clearance (CL_r), especially if they have a more or less pronounced degree of hydrophilicity. For these drugs there is usually a linear relationship between renal function and the ability of the body

to eliminate the drug. The example shown below explains this concept.
This results, from a clinical point of view, in the need to adjust the dosage of these drugs based on a parameter that can correctly estimate the renal function of a subject. This parameter is the creatinine clearance (CL_{cr}).

Example

One study, conducted to assess the pharmacokinetic profile of levofloxacin in patients, showed that the pharmacokinetic data which are obtained in healthy volunteers and published in the literature are hardly comparable with those obtained in patients with diseases. Noteworthy, in patients with impaired renal function, the CL of levofloxacin is reduced, thus resulting in a greater $t_{1/2}$. Since the drug is excreted primarily by the kidneys, the dose should be adapted accordingly: for this reason, the data sheet of medicines containing levofloxacin indicates the dosage adjustments that must be made on the basis of creatinine clearance.

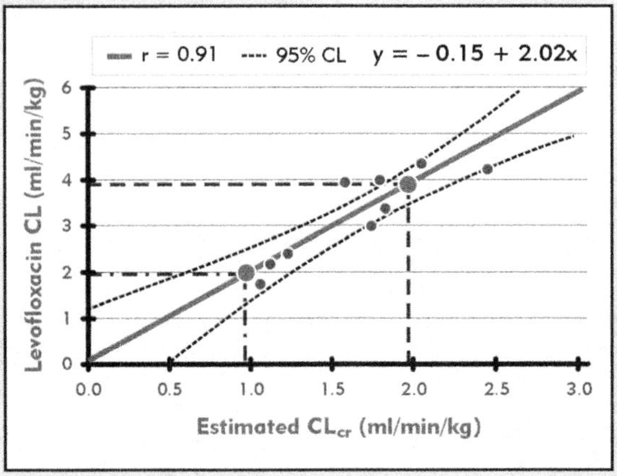

(modified from Pea F, Di Qual E, Cusenza A, Brollo L, Baldassarre M, Furlanut M. Pharmacokinetics and pharmacodynamics of intravenous levofloxacin in patients with early-onset ventilator-associated pneumonia. Clin Pharmacokinet 2003; 42: 589-98)

In this regard, please note that creatinine is an endogenous metabolite coming from the muscle, whose clearance represents a valid surrogate for the extent of glomerular filtration rate because it is filtered in the glomerulus without undergoing any subsequent rearrangement at the tubular level.
The best way to assess CL_{cr} is to measure it directly by collecting the 24-hour urine and a blood sample, and determining the urinary and plasma creatinine concentration according to the following formula:

$$CL_{cr} = \frac{U \times V}{P}$$

where U is the urinary creatinine concentration, V is the 24-hour urine volume, and P is the plasma creatinine concentration.
Indeed, a direct measurement of CL_{cr} is not always feasible in daily clinical practice.
In such cases it becomes extremely useful to calculate creatinine clearance by using the formula that Cockcroft and Gault validated more than 30 years ago and which allows to estimate the extent of glomerular filtration rate of a subject based on few readily available parameters: age, sex, weight, and serum creatinine.
From the Cockcroft and Gault formula, some considerations concerning the CL_{cr} of a given subject can be drawn:

- The higher the value of serum creatinine (S_{cr}) is, the smaller the CL_{cr} will be, considering that this means a decrease in the elimination of creatinine by the kidney.
- Other conditions being equal, CL_{cr} is 15% lower in females than in males, in relation to the smaller size of the kidneys.
- Other conditions being equal, CL_{cr} decreases progressively with age, in relation to glomerulosclerosis.

It therefore seems clear that, for drugs that are excreted by the kidneys, the dose needed to achieve the same therapeutic effect should be modulated taking into account these characteristics. Often, for drugs with predominant renal elimination the dosage adjustments needed on the basis of the patient's CL_{cr}

Antihypertensive	• ACE inhibitors: captopril, enalapril, fosinopril, lisinopril, quinapril, ramipril • Beta-blockers: acebutolol, atenolol, bisoprolol, nadolol • Diuretics: amiloride, spironolactone
Antibiotics	• Carbapenems: ertapenem, imipenem/cilastatin, meropenem • Cephalosporins: cefaclor, cefadroxil, cephalexin, cefamandole, cefazolin, cefepime, cefixime, cefotaxime, cefotetan, cefoxitin, cefpodoxime, cefprozil, cephradine, ceftazidime, ceftibuten, ceftizoxime, cefuroxime • Fluoroquinolones: ciprofloxacin, levofloxacin, norfloxacin, ofloxacin • Macrolides: clarithromycin • Monobactams: aztreonam • Penicillins: amoxicillin (± clavulanate), ampicillin (± sulbactam), carbenicillin, piperacillin (± tazobactam), ticarcillin (± clavulanate) • Sulfonamides: sulfamethoxazole (± trimetoprim)
Antifungal	• Triazoles: fluconazole
Antivirals	• Acyclovir, ganciclovir, valacyclovir, valganciclovir
Statins	• Fluvastatin, pravastatin, rosuvastatin, simvastatin
Other	• Allopurinol, famotidine, gabapentin, metoclopramide, ranitidine

Table XI. Frequently used drugs which need dosage reduction in patients with renal failure.

estimates are reported on the data sheets, and this approach is useful to avoid the risk of toxicity deriving from overexposure. Table XI shows some drugs belonging to the most prescribed therapeutic classes which require dosage adjustments in patients with renal failure.

4.3 Hepatic Failure

Many drugs, especially the lipophilic ones, must be metabolized in order to be eliminated from the body, that is to say they must undergo biotransformation, processes which, by promoting structural changes, may favor their elimination. The organ most commonly involved in these processes is the liver; therefore, it seems logical that in the presence of liver failure, when CL_h is reduced, it may be necessary to reduce the dose of drugs eliminated via the liver or even to avoid their use.

In fact, chronic liver failure, and in particular cirrhosis, is an event that can significantly alter the pharmacokinetics of many drugs, not only with regard to metabolism, but also in any other stage, in relation to the multiple pathophysiological changes that are related to it.

Patients with cirrhosis frequently have portal-hypertensive gastropathy, gastritis and/or ulcers of the gastrointestinal tract that may alter the processes of absorption of orally administered drugs. The most frequent event is a slower oral absorption, resulting in a possible delay in the onset of therapeutic action. In addition, as a result of edema related to hypoalbuminemia and/or ascites related to portal hypertension, there may be a considerable expansion of the extracellular fluid compartment, with an increase of V_d especially for hydrophilic drugs whose distribution is limited only to that compartment (e.g., antibiotics such as beta-lactams, aminoglycosides and glycopeptides).

Surely the most important pharmacokinetic changes that can be found in cirrhotic patients are related to the stage of hepatic metabolism.

Unlike what happens for the assessment of the extent of renal function by measuring the CL_{cr}, no endogenous marker with similar reliability and reproducibility for accurate estimation of patient's liver function exists, so that it becomes difficult to determine what dosage adjustments are necessary in case of organ failure.

For this reason, it was tried to identify some exogenous markers (e.g., indocyanine green, lidocaine-MEGX), but none of these proved to be sufficiently accurate and useful in daily clinical practice in order to predict the kinetic changes of drugs in patients with hepatic failure.

It should also be considered that, as a result of decreased hepatic metabolism, lipophilic drugs can undergo two major types of pharmacokinetic changes:

- Increase in F_{os} in relation to the reduced first-pass effect in the liver.
- Reduction of CL_h because of the comprehensive reduction of hepatic metabolism.

The magnitude of these effects will be different in relation to the hepatic extraction index (E) (Table XII).

For drugs with a high E, which after oral administration in normal conditions undergo an extraction ≥ 60%, the presence of porto-systemic shunts in cirrhotic patients may cause an amount of the portal blood to bypass the liver.

Possible scenarios	Examples of drugs	F_{os} increase in the presence of porto-systemic shunt
Drugs with high hepatic extraction (> 60%)	Fluvastatin, imipramine, isosorbide dinitrate, lovastatin, morphine, nitroglycerin, sertraline	Considerable → Considerable increase in exposure (AUC) → Significant increase in risk of toxicity
Drugs with intermediate hepatic extraction (30-60%)	Amiodarone, amitriptyline, atorvastatin, clomipramine, codeine, erythromycin, pravastatin, simvastatin	Moderate → Moderate increase in exposure (AUC) → Mild increase in risk of toxicity
Drugs with low hepatic extraction (< 30%) and highly protein bound (> 90%)	Clarithromycin, clofibrate, prednisolone, gemfibrozil, tolbutamide	Mild → Slight increase in exposure (AUC) → Very low increase in risk of toxicity
Drugs with low hepatic extraction (< 30%) and poorly protein bound (< 90%)	Alprazolam, bromazepam, carbamazepine, paracetamol, triazolam	Mild → Slight increase in exposure (AUC) → Very low increase in risk of toxicity

Table XII. Changes in the oral bioavailability (F_{os}) of drugs in relation to their degree of hepatic extraction in presence of porto-systemic shunt.

This leads to a significant increase in F_{os},which could result in drug accumulation.
Additionally, considering that hepatic blood flow is frequently reduced in presence of cirrhosis, the CL of these drugs is often decreased. For these reasons, the doses of orally administered drugs with high hepatic extraction (e.g., fluvastatin, imipramine, isosorbide dinitrate, lovastatin, morphine, nitroglycerin, sertraline) must be reduced in patients with cirrhosis.
In this regard, the main difficulty is that often there are no defined guidelines for dosage adjustments of these drugs in patients with cirrhosis; but it is advisable to avoid administration, or otherwise to proceed with small increments of dose according to the clinical outcomes.
For drugs with medium E (30-60%), whose CL depends both on the hepatic flow and on the intrinsic activity of the hepatocytes, in general the F_{os} increase deriving from the porto-systemic shunts is lower than that observed with highly extracted drugs, whereas the decreased hepatic CL requires a significant dose reduction.
For drugs with low E ($<$ 30%), which normally undergo a mild first-pass effect and whose CL is mainly dependent on the intrinsic activity of hepatocytes, the high F_{os} is only moderately increased in course of cirrhosis, whereas the CL may be even significantly decreased in relation to the residual activity of hepatocytes; for this reason the dosage of these drugs should be reduced.
Several studies documented that in cirrhotic patients a progressive reduction in hepatic enzymatic activity occurs in relation with hepatopathy worsening, as documented on the basis of the Child-Pugh score.
For this reason, for the most recently approved drugs there are specific recommendations on dosage adjustments in hepatic impairment (but usually only for Child-Pugh class A and B). Indeed, the kinetic changes depend not only on the severity of the disease, but also on the type of metabolic reaction involved. As a general rule, the oxidative-reductive reactions mediated by CYPs undergo greater reduction than the conjugation ones.

This makes very difficult to standardize the dosage reductions required to avoid overexposure with drugs eliminated predominantly by the liver in patients with cirrhosis.

In the absence of defined recommendations, some authors suggest that, when administering drugs with predominant hepatic elimination, the dose should be equal to 50% of the standard dose for patients with Child-Pugh class A, and to 25% of the standard dose for those with Child-Pugh class B. For patients with Child-Pugh class C, only drugs whose kinetics is unaffected by liver disease should be used.

It should also be noted that in patients with cirrhosis, the predictive value of CL_{cr}, by using the Cockcroft and Gault formula as an endogenous marker of renal glomerular filtration, may be inaccurate, with risk of overstimation of the degree of renal function. In fact, it has been demonstrated that patients with cirrhosis may experience a reduction of the creatinine synthesis and of the skeletal muscle mass. Moreover, in such patients a reduction in the renal blood flow and in the extent of glomerular filtration rate has been occasionally documented, even in the absence of ascites. For these reasons, especially in severely ill patients, it is recommended to measure creatinine clearance in order to accurately assess renal function and to allow the choice of the most appropriate dose of renally cleared drugs.

Child-Pugh classification

The Child-Pugh (or Child-Pugh Turcotte) score is a classification system that enables the assessment of disease severity in patients with chronic hepatitis, based on the results of laboratory tests (bilirubin, PT, albumin) and physical findings (presence of hepatic encephalopathy and/or of ascites). To each variable a score is assigned, the total of which defines the severity of the disease. Higher scores are associated with more severe disease and more severe impairment of liver function. Based on the mixed score, three Child-Pugh classes can be defined:

- A: score = 5-6
- B: score = 7-9
- C: score > 9

4.4 The Critically Ill Patient

The critically ill patient often presents a number of pathophysiological and/or iatrogenic situations that alter significantly the pharmacokinetics of many drugs. For this reason, doses that are used in this context can sometimes be very different from those that are generally used in stable patients.

The most relevant pathophysiological mechanisms that may more frequently affect the kinetic profile of the drugs in the critically ill patients are the changes in the extracellular fluids content and/or in the degree of functionality of the excretory organs (kidneys and/or liver). These pathophysiological situations will lead to changes in the drug V_d and CL, respectively, whose relevance will vary in relation to the physicochemical characteristics of the given drug.

In fact, the intra- and inter-individual variability of pharmacokinetics in the critically ill patients concerns primarily the hydrophilic drugs rather than the lipophilic ones, because the former are affected to a greater extent by the changes of both the extracellular fluid content and the renal function.

For example, for the hydrophilic drugs the presence of a large pleural effusion (e.g., 3 l) may result in a significant increase

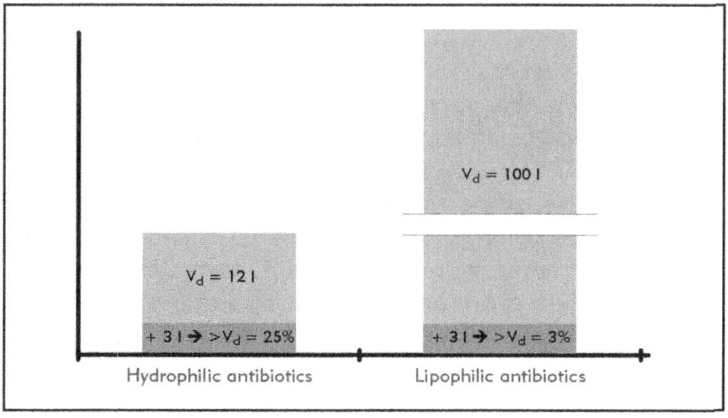

Figure 33. V_d and increased extracellular fluids.

in their total V_d with consequent dilution (Figure 33), since these drugs, due to their limited distribution in the extracellular space, have a very low total V_d (approximately 12-15 l under normal conditions).
By contrast, for lipophilic drugs the increase in V_d will be less relevant because these drugs, by having high V_d (often higher than 70-100 l) and by accumulating within cells which may act as a reservoir, will be affected to a lesser extent by the dilution resulting from the expansion of extracellular fluid thanks to the redistribution from the intracellular to the extracellular space that will occur.
Likewise, hydrophilic and/or moderately lipophilic drugs which are excreted mainly in unchanged form by the kidneys, may undergo considerable daily fluctuations in plasma concentrations due to significant changes in their CL whenever the renal function fluctuates, a situation often in dynamic evolution in the critically ill patients.
In contrast, lipophilic drugs that are metabolized by the liver undergo only small or moderate changes in their pharmacokinetic profile due to changes in renal function, but may undergo significant changes as a result of modifications of liver function. However, unlike renal function, daily fluctuations of liver function are uncommon even in the case of the critically ill patients, so that considerable reductions in elimination occur only in the presence of severe liver diseases (e.g., hepatic cirrhosis, acute hepatitis) that are able to significantly reduce liver blood flow and/or its metabolic activity. Therefore, usually there are no significant fluctuations in plasma concentrations of these drugs in the same patient in the brief period.
Generally speaking, the drugs that are more frequently affected by significant pharmacokinetic variations in the critically ill patients are represented by certain classes of hydrophilic antibiotics, namely beta-lactams, aminoglycosides and glycopeptides. Splitting antibiotics into two categories according to their physicochemical properties, hydrophilic and lipophilic agents, can be very useful to better understand how the pathophysiological processes may alter their plasma profile (Table XIII).

Hydrophilic antibiotics	Lipophilic antibiotics
• Unable to cross the plasma membrane by passive diffusion • Low volume of distribution (< 12-20 l) • Eliminated mainly unchanged by the kidney • Inactive against intracellular pathogens	• Able to cross plasma membranes by passive diffusion • High volume of distribution (> 40-70 l) • Eliminated mainly by metabolism, often by the liver • Active against intracellular pathogens

Table XIII. Physicochemical characteristics of antibiotics.

Hydrophilic antibiotics, including beta-lactams, aminoglycosides and glycopeptides, are characterized by the inability to cross the membrane of the eukaryotic cell by passive diffusion, which means that:

- From a pharmacokinetic point of view, they have a low volume of distribution (total V_d < 12-20 l) due to an exclusively extracellular distribution which is limited to the plasma and to the interstitial spaces of tissues, and an almost complete renal elimination in unchanged form.
- From a pharmacodynamic point of view, they are inactive against intracellular pathogens (for example, *Legionella pneumophila, Mycoplasma pneumoniae*).

By contrast, the lipophilic antibiotics, including macrolides, fluoroquinolones, rifampin, tetracycline, chloramphenicol, and oxazolidinones, are characterized by the ability of passive diffusion through the membrane of eukaryotic cells, which means that:

- From a pharmacokinetic point of view, they exhibit a higher volume of distribution (total V_d > 40-70 l) as a result of intracellular penetration, and an elimination by metabolism, frequently by the liver.
- From a pharmacodynamic point of view, they have good activity against intracellular pathogens (for example, *Legionella pneumophila, Mycoplasma pneumoniae*).

Indeed, within the group of lipophilic antibiotics, some notable exceptions exist. Levofloxacin and ciprofloxacin are moderately

lipophilic fluoroquinolones that, while penetrating into the cells, are excreted predominantly as unchanged form by the kidneys. Azithromycin is an azalide classified in the macrolide group which, although considerably lipophilic, is eliminated as unchanged form almost exclusively through the biliary route.
Table XIV summarizes the main pathophysiological and iatrogenic conditions which may change the pharmacokinetic profile of the antibiotics in the critically ill patients and their relevance in conditioning the need for a change of the drug dosing regimens.
There are several pathophysiological situations that, by causing an increase in the V_d, can cause a reduction in the concentration of hydrophilic antibiotics in plasma and in the extracellular fluids. For example, during sepsis or trauma extensive expansion of extracellular fluid can occur as a result of increased capillary permeability promoted by the endothelial leakage and by the significant reduction of intravascular oncotic pressure due

Changes in extracellular fluids	Changes in renal function	
Increase	Increase	Decrease
• Edema • Effusion in sierous cavities • Fluid load • Hypoalbuminemia	• Hyperdynamic sepsis • 3rd degree burns > 30% of body surface • Hemodynamically active drugs (dopamine, dobutamine, furosemide) • Acute leukemia • Hypoalbuminemia	• Renal failure • Dialysis
• **> Vd and antibiotic dilution** • **> LD of hydrophilic antibiotics**	• **> renal CL of antibiotic** • **> MD of antibiotics eliminated by the kidney**	• **< renal CL of antibiotic** • **< MD of antibiotics eliminated by the kidney**

Table XIV. Pathophysiological conditions that alter the pharmacokinetic profile of antibiotics.

to hypoalbuminemia. This collection of fluids in the interstitial spaces of tissues is called "the third space phenomenon" and may have important consequences if the critically ill patients are treated with standard doses of antibiotics. Therefore, in order to ensure adequate exposure, it would be appropriate to begin therapy with an increased LD. Similarly, during hyperdynamic sepsis or co-administration of hemodynamically active drugs, there may be an increase in renal plasma flow, which results in an increase of CL_r of hydrophilic antibiotics, with the consequent need to increase the MD. In contrast, in the presence of renal failure, when CL_r decreases, it will be necessary to reduce the MD of hydrophilic antibiotics. In this regard it must be considered that, similarly to what was previously reported for the stable patients, even in the critically ill ones it is often possible to estimate correctly the extent of glomerular filtration rate by using the Cockcroft and Gault formula.
However, since creatinine is a product of muscle metabolism, it should not be overlooked that this formula cannot be applied to reliably estimate CL_{cr} in the case of persons who are immobilized for a long time (e.g., paraplegics or tetraplegics, or individuals who are bedridden for more than three to four weeks). In such cases, for a correct assessment of glomerular filtration rate, it is recommended to measure directly the CL_{cr} by using the 24-hour urine collection according to the formula:

$$CL_{cr} = \frac{U \times V}{P}$$

where U is the mean concentration of creatinine in the urine over 24 hours, V is the volume of urine over 24 hours and P is the plasma concentration of creatinine.

5 PHARMACOKINETICS AND PHARMACEUTICAL TECHNOLOGY

From what has already been described in the previous chapters, it is clear that the efficacy and the tolerability of a drug are the consequence of the concentrations that it achieves in the various body districts in relation to its pharmacokinetic characteristics.
If the intrinsic pharmacokinetics of a given drug is not particularly suitable, through the pharmaceutical technology it is possible to produce structural changes, in order to improve its pharmacokinetics. This can be useful, for example, in the case of drugs that are characterized by a low therapeutic index and are therefore burdened by a high toxicological risk. In such cases, the active drug can be embedded within particular vectors that primarily acts as carriers of the drug to the site of action by reducing the ubiquitous tissue accumulation and thus the risk of toxicity. This approach is used, for example, for lipid formulations of some antineoplastic drugs and of some antifungal drugs.
In other cases, the pharmacokinetics of a drug may be particularly unsuitable with regard to the patient compliance to the dosage regimens proposed with the therapy. This may occur, for example, in the case of drugs that originally have a very short $t_{1/2}$, so that the patient is required to take the drugs several times throughout the day. In this case, technology can provide some helpful tools in implementing pharmaceutical formulations structured in such a way as to allow a progressive release of the drug: the so-called depot preparations or controlled release preparations.
Finally, the pharmaceutical technology can also enable to change the original structure of a drug in order to improve its F_{os}. In this case, the drug may be linked to a molecule that is

normally easily absorbed by the gastrointestinal tract, such as an aminoacid which is absorbed by means of specific enteric transporters, and, that once having reached the blood, is then rapidly converted to its active form. In this case the modified drug is defined as prodrug. Below are reported three examples that illustrate these specific situations.

5.1 Liposomal Formulations

In recent years, the pharmaceutical technology has provided fundamental support to allow an improvement in the safety of certain drugs with low therapeutic index through the development of the so-called liposomal formulations. This approach is used, for example, for some chemotherapeutic drugs in order to reduce their toxicity (e.g., nephrotoxicity of amphotericin B among antifungal drugs, and cardiotoxicity of daunorubicin and doxorubicin among antineoplastic drugs).

In these cases, the main purpose of the pharmaceutical technology is to allow the active principle to remain stably incorporated into the preparation during transport throughout the body, being then released as close as possible to the site of action (e.g., the site of infection or of malignancy). In this way, the ubiquitous tissue distribution of the drug is limited, as well as, consequently, the contact with the normal cells of the body. From a pharmacokinetic point of view, this corresponds to a considerable reduction in the V_d of the liposomal formulation of the drug compared to the free one, with a consequent increase in the C_{max} and in the plasma AUC. As an example, we report a comparison between the pharmacokinetic characteristics of an antineoplastic agent, daunorubicin, in the free form and in the liposomal one (Table XV).

This comparison shows that, under the same dose, liposomal formulation allows to limit the tissue distribution and consequently the risk of toxicity. Indeed, the stability of the liposomal formulation in the bloodstream depends on the structural characteristics of its components: it is greater for those liposomes

	C_{max} (µg/ml)	V_d (l/m^2)	AUC (µg x h/ml)	CL (l/h/m^2)
Free daunorubicin 60 mg/m^2	0.80	1,297	0.63	199.8
Liposomal daunorubicin 60 mg/m^2	23.64	2.88	456.27	0.47

Table XV. Main pharmacokinetic parameters of free and liposomal daunorubicin.

AUC = area under the plasma concentration-time curve, CL = clearance, C_{max} = maximum plasmatic concentration, V_d = volume of distribution

containing phospholipids with low degree of unsaturation which have transition temperature (i.e., the temperature at which the prepared liposomal naturally tends to collapse, releasing its contents) above the body temperature, and cholesterol. The remarkable stability of the circulating liposomal formulation of daunorubicin did not affect its usefulness, however, since it has been shown that liposomes are able to accumulate passively in the tumor site, due to the increased permeability of the newly formed vessels.

5.2 Controlled Release or Depot Formulations

Sometimes intrinsic pharmacokinetic characteristics of a given drug do not appear to be particularly suitable from a clinical point of view. For example, in the case of drugs that should be used during chronic therapy, a very short $t_{1/2}$ may cause the need to use multiple daily doses (e.g., every 4-6 hours) with obvious consequences for the patient compliance. In such circumstances, pharmaceutical technology provides help, by allowing the use of controlled release or depot formulations. These formulations are structured in such a way as to allow the gradual release of the active drug from the site of administration (e.g., gut, if oral; muscle, if intramuscular; skin, if transdermal) to the systemic circulation. In such a way a situation similar to that observed with frequent administration of small doses of the original compound may be obtained. In the case of oral formulations, sometimes the structure is much like an onion, in which just shell after shell immediate-release and slow-release drug are applied. In some cases, in formulations for parenteral use, the active drug is complexed with substances that slow down the elimination, as is the case for benzathine-benzylpenicillin which, after intramuscular administration, progressively releases, through hydrolysis, active benzylpenicillin.

Of course, regardless of the pharmaceuticals technology used, controlled release formulations cause a significant change in the pharmacokinetic behavior of the active drug: in many cases, t_{max} is delayed and C_{max} appears to be reduced, whereas AUC is increased and $t_{1/2}$ prolonged due to a reduction in CL (Figure 34).

From a pharmacological clinical point of view, controlled release formulations, given the longer residence time in the body, are useful for those drugs requiring the maintenance of a constant

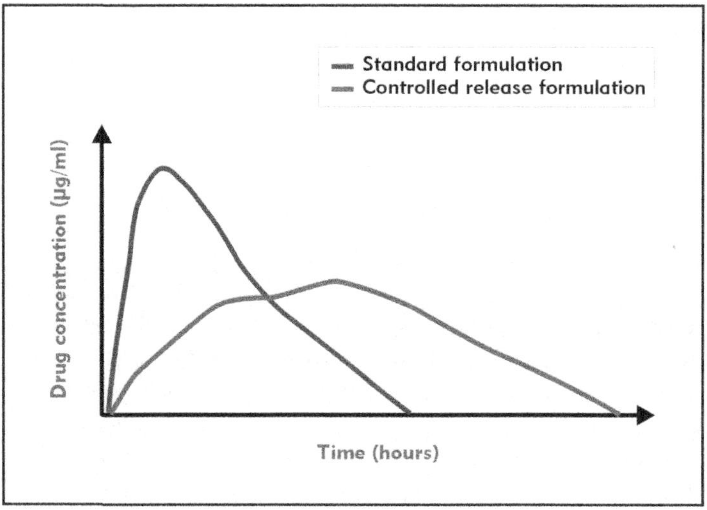

Figure 34. Comparison of the plasma concentration-time profile of a drug in standard formulation vs. controlled release formulation.

action during the whole day, as is the case with antihypertensive drugs (verapamil) or antiasthmatic ones (e.g., theophylline). On the other hand, considering t_{max} prolongation and C_{max} decrease, their use is usually unsuitable for drugs requiring a rapid onset of action.

5.3 Prodrugs

Drugs that are used in therapy are usually administered in an already active form. In some cases, however, mainly in order to enhance their pharmacokinetic behavior, it can be helpful to use drugs that are activated into the body after having been administered: these are the so-called prodrugs. In recent years, the use of prodrugs was mainly done to increase the F_{os} of certain substances. For example, antiviral drugs such as acyclovir and ganciclovir are characterized by very poor F_{os}, with the consequent need of administering oral doses several-folds higher than those administered by the intravenous route. Recently, the complexation of these antiviral drugs with the aminoacid

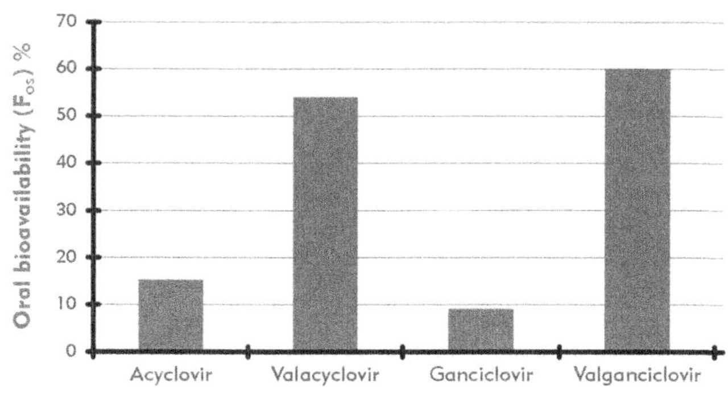

Figure 35. Comparison of the value of F_{os} between acyclovir and ganciclovir and their prodrugs, valacyclovir and valganciclovir.

valine has led to two prodrugs, valacyclovir and valganciclovir, whose F_{os} turns out to be significantly higher (Figure 35).
In fact, these prodrugs are absorbed in the intestine by means of the peptide carrier-mediated transport and subsequently hydrolyzed by intestinal and liver esterases with immediate release of the active drug. Thanks to this, daily dosage can be reduced, both in terms of the amount of the single dose and in that of the number of the daily doses, thus obtaining a therapeutic effect similar to that achievable after intravenous administration.

6 PHARMACOKINETICS AND PHARMACOGENETICS

Pharmacogenetics is the science that studies the variability of drug response in relation to genetic factors involved in the processes that are responsible for the pharmacokinetic fate of and/or for the mechanism of action of a drug in the body.

This chapter will briefly outline pharmacogenetics principles that can cause a considerable interindividual pharmacokinetic variability. This variability appears to be related to the existence of genetic polymorphisms. In other words, this is due to the fact that some of the genes encoding for enzymes responsible for phase I or II metabolism may have allelic variants.

These variants are able to encode for different molecular isoforms of the same protein and, in most cases, they depend on single nucleotide polymorphisms (SNPs), which determine the production of isoforms that differ each other for a single aminoacid.

The variations in the DNA sequence of genes encoding for metabolizing enzymes can cause considerable phenotypic differences in the expressivity and in the activity of an enzyme.

Individuals who have two allellic variants that encode for the normal enzyme function are identified as extensive metabolizers (EMs), whereas those who have two allelic variants that encode for a modified enzyme, inactive or absent, are called poor metabolizers (PMs). In some cases, it may happen that some individuals have multiple copies of the gene encoding for normal enzyme activity, so that the metabolizing capacity will be considerably increased, and these subjects will be defined as ultrarapid metabolizers (UMs).

These genetically predetermined differences in the expressiveness and in the activity of the enzymatic packages responsible for drug metabolization, by affecting to a different extent drug clearance, may be responsible for a wide interindividual variability in AUC, even when standard doses adjusted per body weight are used.

Figure 36 shows some examples of the variability in plasma exposure which may occur with the administration of a standard dose of a drug that is substrate of the polymorphic enzyme with respect to its phenotypic expression.

The standard dose will achieve adequate exposure in terms of AUC only in the EM, who may theoretically benefit from the

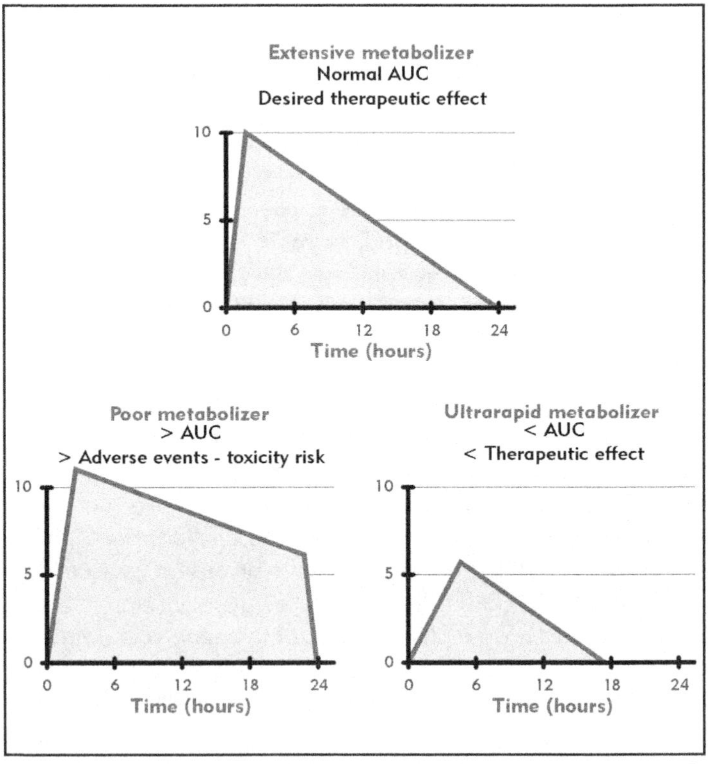

Figure 36. Polymorphic metabolism and variability of exposure to standard dose.

desired therapeutic effect. In the PM, however, it will cause over-exposure, thus leading to a higher incidence of adverse effects and increased risk of toxicity. In contrast, in the UM drug exposure after standard dose is considerably lower than desired, so that the therapeutic response will be only partial.
It is also interesting to note that the incidence of polymorphisms of genes encoding for metabolizing enzymes can sometimes vary even considerably in relation to race and ethnicity. Although many genetic polymorphisms exist, indeed only some have clinically relevant consequences in terms of drug metabolism.
This occurs more frequently when the following two conditions coexist: the involved metabolic pathway is the only metabolic pathway of the given drug, and the drug is characterized by a low therapeutic index, i.e., the range between the effective dose and the toxic dose is relatively small. As an example, we describe some peculiar situations of considerable clinical interest.

6.1 Polymorphism of Phase I Enzymes

With regard to the phase I enzymes, clinically relevant genetic polymorphisms are mainly related to three isoforms of the CYP450: CYP2D6, CYP2C19, and CYP2C9. By contrast, the CYP3A4 isoform, the most quantitatively important in terms of drug metabolism, does not seem to have clinically relevant genetic polymorphisms.

6.1.1 CYP2D6 Polymorphism

The gene encoding for CYP2D6 is one of the most interesting polymorphic genes from a pharmacological point of view and has been extensively studied. Poor metabolizers, who represents on average 5-10% of the population, are carriers of two allelic variants that have no function; the UM individuals, who correspond to 1-10% of the population, are carriers of active genes in duplicate or multiple copies. It follows therefore that, globally, 5-20% of patients being treated with standard doses of a drug that is a CYP2D6 substrate could be potentially at risk of toxicity due to overexposure or, conversely, at risk of treatment failure due to underexposure, depending whether they are PMs or UMs.

The best-studied examples in the literature are related to tricyclic antidepressants (amitriptyline, clomipramine, desipramine, imipramine, nortriptyline). In particular, for nortriptyline (Table XVI) it was observed that for CYP2D6 extensive metabolizers, who represent the majority of patients (approximately 80-94%), the dose required to reach the therapeutically effective C_{ss} (200-600 nmol/l) is of 75-150 mg/day. On the other hand in PMs, in order to get the same exposure, lower doses are sufficient (20-30 mg/day), while in the UM considerably higher doses (300-500 mg/day or more) are required.

In relation to these considerations, it is necessary to assume that CYP2D6 poor metabolizers may have a greater incidence of adverse events during therapy with standard doses of tricyclic antidepressants (e.g., tachycardia, constipation, urinary retention), whereas, on the other hand, ultrarapid metabolizers may not obtain a good control of the depressive state.

Similarly, it is interesting to note that the same potential problem may occur with some antiarrhythmic drugs that are substrates of CYP2D6, such as some beta-blockers (metoprolol, propranolol, timolol), flecainide, propafenone and mexiletine.

	Poor metabolizer (5-10%)	Extensive metabolizer (80-94%)	Ultrarapid metabolizer (1-10%)
Dose of nortriptyline to achieve therapeutic C_{ss} of 200-600 nmol/l (mg/day)	20-30	75-150	≥ 300-500

Table XVI. Dose of nortriptyline needed to achieve therapeutic effective concentrations in relation to the different CYP2D6 phenotypes.

6.1.2 | CYP2C19 Polymorphism

The frequency of CYP2C19 poor metabolizers is particularly high in the Asian ethnic group (on average 15-20%), whereas it is much lower in Caucasians (2-3%).
The polymorphism of CYP2C19 may be of particular clinical relevance with regard to the variability of exposure to certain proton pump inhibitors (e.g., lansoprazole, omeprazole, and pantoprazole) and diazepam.
For example, it was found that for both omeprazole and lansoprazole, the AUC can be up to 4-15 times higher in PMs than in EMs after a single dose of the drug.
It is interesting to note that some authors have shown that in CYP2C19 PM patients suffering from peptic ulcer who were co-treated with omeprazole and clarithromycin, there was higher healing rate than in EMs, probably related to more potent suppression of the production of chloridric acid.
Similarly, with regard to diazepam it has been shown that exposure can be up to six times higher in PMs than in EMs, thus causing a more prolonged sedation.

6.1.3 | CYP2C9 Polymorphism

The polymorphism of CYP2C9 may be particularly relevant in determining a wide interindividual pharmacokinetic variability in patients receiving oral anticoagulation therapy with warfarin.
In fact, CYP2C9 is involved in the metabolism of the levorotatory isomer of this drug (S-warfarin), which is the main responsible of the anticoagulant effect of warfarin, being about five times more potent than the dextrorotatory one (R-warfarin, a CYP3A4 substrate). Recent studies have shown that 20-30% of patients on warfarin therapy, being CYP2C9 PMs (1-7% homozygotes, 14-28% heterozygotes), may have a more or less reduced metabolism of this drug in comparison with the normal standard. These patients, with larger drug exposure, may therefore be at increased risk of bleeding during treatment with standard

doses. The importance of this aspect is underlined by the fact that the Food and Drug Administration recently decided to fund several research projects with the aim of being able to identify warfarin dosing regimens that can be modulated according to this situation.

6.2 Polymorphism of Phase II Enzymes

The most studied genetic polymorphisms in relation to the activity of phase II metabolizing enzymes are mainly the N-acetyltransferase (NAT2) and the thiopurine methyltransferase (TPMT).

6.2.1 NAT2 Polymorphism

The process of metabolism of isoniazid by acetyltransferase encoded by the NAT2 gene is one of the first studied examples of genetically predetermined clinically relevant differences for phase II enzymes.

In this respect two different classes of subjects were identified: the rapid acetylators, who are supplied with a normal functioning enzyme, and slow acetylators who, in contrast, have a reduced metabolizing capacity.

Even for such a genetic polymorphism, similarly to what happens for other genes encoding drug-metabolizing enzymes, there is a wide variability of expression within a population in relation to ethnicity: the proportion of slow acetylators is in fact of about 40-70% in Caucasians, but drops to around 20% in the Asian ethnic group.

Some authors have hypothesized that in slow acetylators the lack of acetyltransferase activity, by causing an increased formation of highly reactive intermediate metabolites (hydrazine) by means of other metabolic pathways, can be correlated with the higher incidence of hepatotoxicity observed during antituberculosis treatment with standard doses of isoniazid.

6.2.2 TPMT Polymorphism

TPMT is an enzyme responsible for the metabolism of thiopurine antimetabolites, azathioprine and thiopurine, used for the treatment of certain hematologic malignancies. This enzyme, which is usually present in high amounts in red blood cells and other tissues, may have a low level of activity or may be completely inactive in relation to a genetic polymorphism that encodes for a variant that differs by two aminoacids.

The presence of this deficient variant, whose frequency varies according to ethnicity (1 every 300 in Caucasians, 1 every 2,500 in Asians), can cause an increased bone marrow toxicity during therapy with standard doses of thiopurine.

In view of this, phenotyping tests have been developed (evaluation of the expression of TPMT in red blood cells), as well as genotyping ones (assessment of the allelic variants of TPMT), in order to individualize antineoplastic therapy with thiopurines in relation to the state of activity of TPMT. This last example is one of the first attempts to exploit the knowledge of pharmacogenetics to optimize the pharmacokinetic exposure to a given drug.

In relation to the previously reported data, and with the progressive improvement of knowledge, it is conceivable that in the near future, genotyping and/or phenotyping tests may be helpful, at least in some cases, in an attempt to improve the effectiveness of, and to prevent the onset of adverse reactions to drugs that are substrates of metabolizing enzymes encoded by polymorphic genes.

7 PHARMACOKINETICS AND PHARMACODYNAMICS

The therapeutic effect of a drug may be considered the result of an integration between the pharmacodynamics (**the science that studies the mechanism of action of drugs**) and the pharmacokinetics (**the science that studies the movement of drugs within a living organism**). This correlation, which is precisely defined as **pharmacokinetic-pharmacodynamic** relationship (PK/PD), is aimed at ensuring the maintenance of therapeutically effective concentrations of the drug at the site of action. The field of antimicrobial therapy is one of those in which the most significant progress in this direction has been made in recent years.

7.1 Pharmacokinetic-pharmacodynamic (PK/PD) Relationships in Antibiotic Therapy

The fundamental prerequisite for appropriate treatment consists in choosing an antibiotic with an appropriate spectrum of activity including the etiologic agent responsible for the infection. Although this condition is necessary, however, not always it is sufficient to ensure the patient's healing and the microbiological eradication of the infection. In fact, these depend also on the appropriateness of the chosen dosing regimen (in terms of single dose and frequency of administration) that should necessarily be different in relation to the various ways in which the antibiotics exert their antibacterial activity.
Over the last fifteen years, the study of PK/PD relationships of antibiotics allowed to demonstrate that these drugs can carry out their antibacterial activity in a time-dependent or in a concentration-dependent manner (Table XVII).

Time-dependent antibiotics	Concentration-dependent antibiotics
Beta-lactams: • Carbapenems • Cephalosporins • Monobactams • Penicillins Glycopeptides Natural macrolides Oxazolidinones	Aminoglycosides Fluoroquinolones Lipopeptides

Table XVII. Classification of antibiotics according to type of antibacterial activities.

Time-dependent antibiotics, including beta-lactams, glycopeptides, natural macrolides, and oxazolidinones, present as major pharmacodynamic determinant of their effect the time during which plasma concentrations of the antibiotic are maintained above the minimum inhibitory concentration (MIC) of the patho-

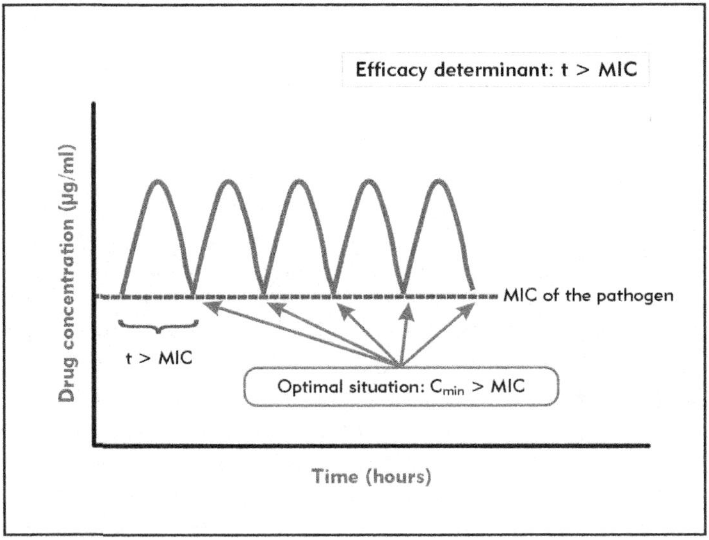

Figure 37. Effectiveness of time-dependent antibiotics.

gen (t > MIC). Although a t > MIC of at least 50-60% of the dosing interval may be sufficient to achieve good clinical response in immunocompetent subjects, conversely a t > MIC of 100% of the dosing interval, or a minimum plasma concentration (C_{min}) just before drug re-administration greater than the MIC of the pathogen (C_{min} > MIC) (Figure 37) are required in order to ensure optimal exposure in immunocompromised patients and/or for the treatment of more severe infections occurring in the critically ill patients.
These antibiotics are defined as time-dependent because their effectiveness depends only slightly on the peak concentrations reached, since the highest antibacterial activity can be obtained already at concentrations of about 4-5 times the MIC. In fact, any further increase in concentration to values that are equal, for example, to tens or hundreds of times the MIC does not in any way increase the effectiveness of time-dependent antibiotics, but may result in increased toxicity.
Taking into consideration these characteristics, it is clear that, from a pharmacokinetic point of view, the most beneficial reg-

Frequency of administration	Antibiotics
Every 4 hours	Ampicillin Oxacillin
Every 6 hours	Amoxicillin ± clavulanic acid (IV) Piperacillin ± tazobactam Vancomycin
Every 8 hours	Amoxicillin ± clavulanic acid (os) Cefepime Cefotaxime Ceftazidime
Every 12 hours	Clarithromycin Linezolid
Every 24 hours	Ceftriaxone Teicoplanin

Table XVIII. **Frequency of administration of some time-dependent antibiotics.**

imen in order to maintain C_{min} > MIC is the multi-fractionation of the daily dose, which should be more frequent the shorter the $t_{1/2}$ of a given drug is (Table XVIII).
In addition, continuous intravenous infusion (CI) may be a helpful tool to improve the performance of time-dependent antibiotics, since, under the same total daily dose, it allows to obtain higher values of C_{min} > MIC, due to the fact that, in this case, C_{min} coincides with the C_{ss} (Figure 38).

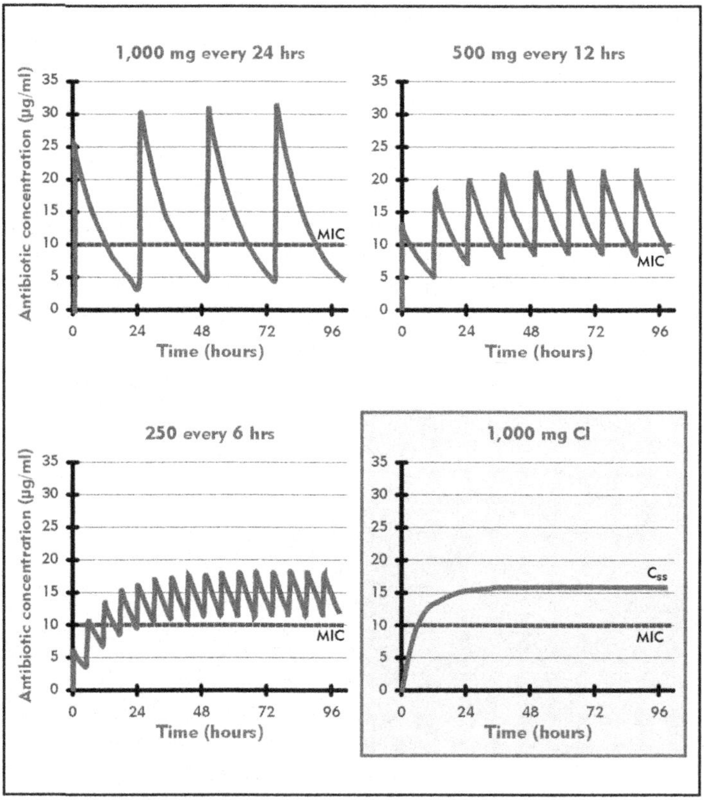

Figure 38. Changes in plasma concentration profile of the same single daily dose of medication according to different modes of administration; continuous infusion is the optimal way for time-dependent antibiotics.

The concentration-dependent antibiotics, including fluoroquinolones, aminoglycosides and lipopeptides, are characterized by the fact that their antibacterial activity increases progressively with increasing concentration, theoretically, without ever reaching a plateau.
The major pharmacodynamic determinants of their antibacterial activity are the ratio between maximum plasma concentration and the MIC (C_{max}/MIC) and that between the area under the plasma concentration-time curve (AUC) and the MIC (AUC/MIC). In fact, several studies showed that threshold values of C_{max}/MIC > 10-12 may ensure good clinical response and prevent the onset of resistance.
As far as AUC/MIC ratio is concerned, it is believed that different threshold values are required for Gram-positive species and Gram-negative ones, probably in relation to their different extent of virulence and of pathogenicity: AUC/MIC values > 100-125 are required for Gram-negative species, whereas values > 30-50 seem to be sufficient for Gram-positive ones (Figure 39).

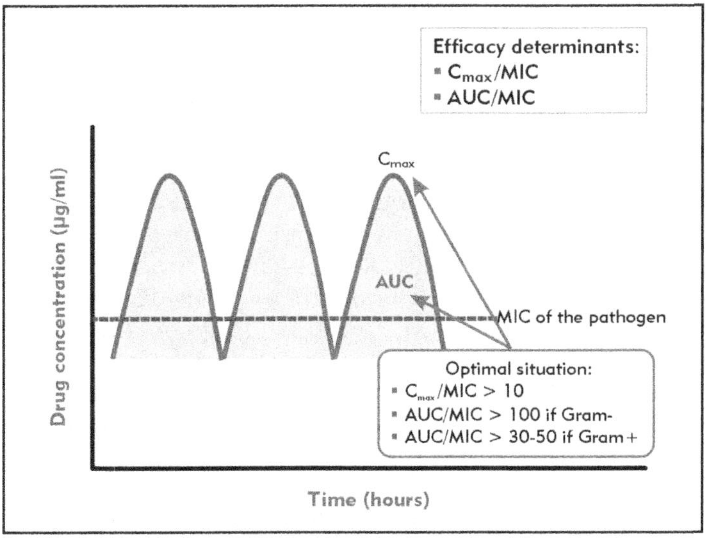

Figure 39. Efficacy of concentration-dependent antibiotics.

Considering that AUC = dose/CL, it is clear that the dose fractioning does not affect the value of AUC/MIC because, under the same total daily dose, the value of this ratio will be the same in the same patient, regardless of the mode in which the dose was fractionated.
On the contrary, under the same total daily dose, the route of administration certainly affects the value of the C_{max} /MIC ratio, since C_{max} will be higher the lower the dose fractioning is. Therefore, aminoglycosides, fluoroquinolones and lipopeptides should be administered once daily or twice daily, depending on their pharmacokinetic characteristics and on their tolerability (Figure 40).
Regarding this aspect, it must be remembered that aminoglycosides, unlike in the past, should be administered once daily (e.g., gentamicin, tobramycin, and netilmicin 3-5 mg/kg every 24 hours, amikacin 15 mg/kg every 24 hours) irrespective of their plasma half-life elimination being relatively short (2.5 to 4 hours) and of their known nephrotoxicity.
This can be explained by considering that these antibiotics have a valid post-antibiotic effect (PAE, that is the persistent suppression of bacterial growth even when the antibiotic concentrations fall below the MIC of the pathogen) against most of the sensitive bacterial species, both Gram-positive and Gram-negative, which on average lasts some hours. In addition, several studies have shown that once daily dose of aminoglycosides does not increase nephrotoxicity or ototoxicity. This can be explained by considering that aminoglycosides are water-soluble drugs whose penetration into the renal tubular cells and the cochlear cells does not occur by passive diffusion, but is mediated by carriers. Since this transport is characterized by a saturative kinetics, giving the entire dose at one time can probably saturate the transport system by allowing, in relation to the short $t_{1/2}$, the elimination of most of the drug by the kidney before the carrier will become available again.
In contrast, fluoroquinolones are administered once or twice daily in relation to their plasma elimination half-life. For example, ciprofloxacin, having a half-life of about 4-5 hours, is

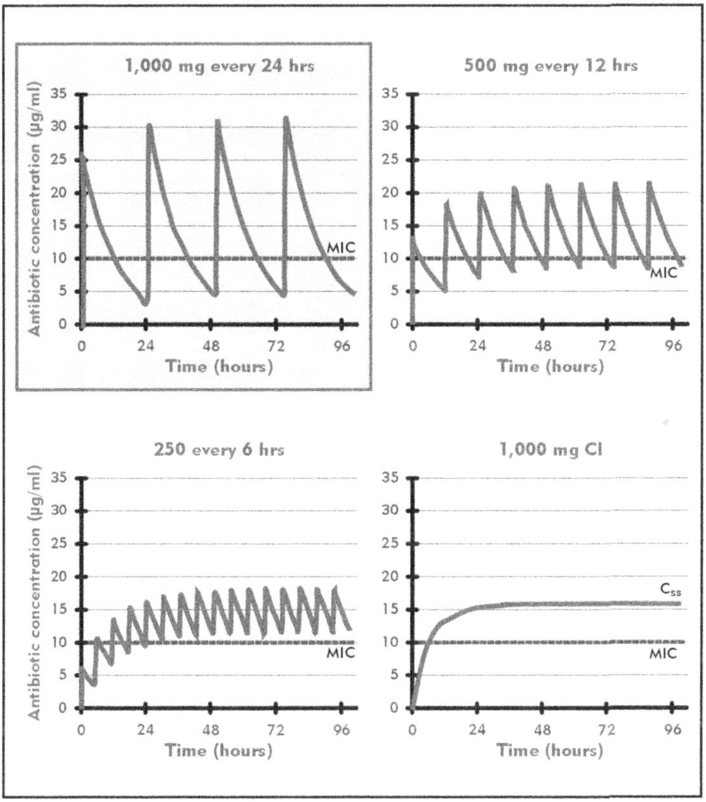

Figure 40. Changes in plasma concentration profile of the same single daily dose of medication according to different modes of administration. The single dose is the optimal way for concentration-dependent antibiotics activities.

administered twice daily, whereas levofloxacin and moxifloxacin, which have $t_{1/2}$ of 7 and 12 hours, respectively, are administered once daily. However fluoroquinolones, unlike aminoglycosides, being lipid soluble drugs for their intrinsic physicochemical properties, are able to cross cell membranes by passive diffusion and, therefore, their tolerance may be reduced when the single daily dose is excessively high, as their penetration naturally in-

Frequency of administration	Antibiotics
Every 24 hours	Amikacin, daptomycin, gentamicin, levofloxacin, moxifloxacin, netilmicin, tobramycin
Every 12 hours	Ciprofloxacin

Table XIX. Frequency of administration of some concentration-dependent antibiotics.

creases depending on the concentration gradient. For this reason, when it is necessary to increase the efficacy of fluoroquinolones, it is preferred to intensify, beyond a certain level of a single dose, the frequency of administration, which allows an increase in the AUC/MIC ratio (Table XIX).

7.2 Pharmacokinetic-pharmacodynamic (PK/PD) Relationships in Antifungal Therapy

Finally, a brief look at PK/PD correlations for antifungal drugs. Similarly to what has been widely demonstrated for antibiotics, recent studies have shown that taking into account whether activity is dose-dependent or time-dependent may be fundamental even for the adequate therapeutic use of antifungal drugs. The triazoles (fluconazole, itraconazole, posaconazole and voriconazole) and flucytosine are time-dependent drugs, and therefore their efficacy depends primarily on t > MIC (Figure 41).
In contrast, polyenes (amphotericin B) and echinocandins (anidulafungin, caspofungin and micafungin) have concentration-dependent activities, and therefore the major determinant of their efficacy is the ratio between maximum concentration and MIC (C_{max}/MIC) (Figure 42).
These observations suggest that fractioning the daily dose according to drug $t_{1/2}$ is the most suitable mode of administering the triazoles and flucytosine (Table XX), whereas once-daily administration must be pursued with polyenes and echinocandins (Table XXI).

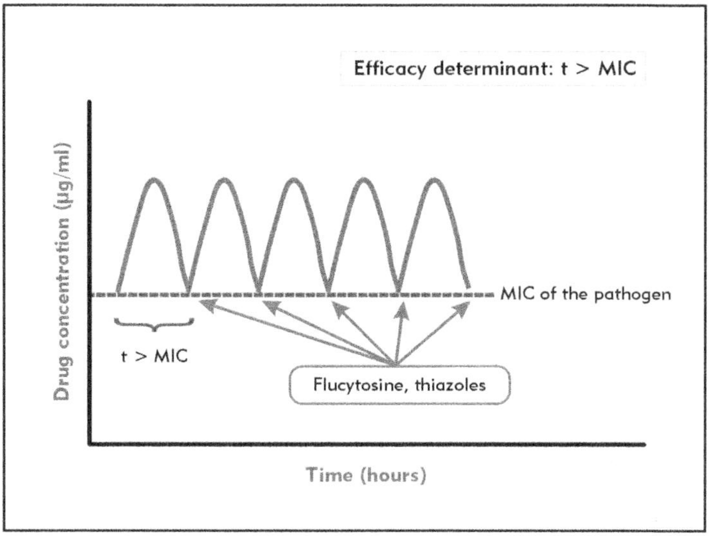

Figure 41. Efficacy of time-dependent antifungal agents.

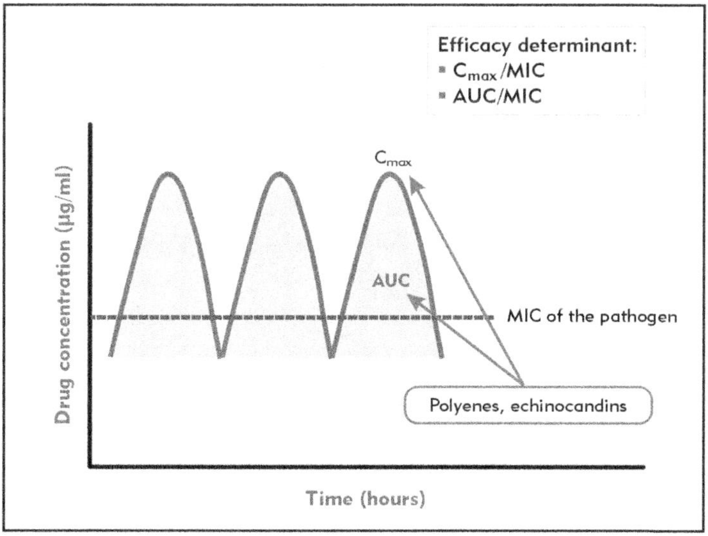

Figure 42. Efficacy of concentration-dependent antifungal agents.

Frequency of administration	Antifungal agents
Every 6 hours	Flucytosine, posaconazole
Every 12 hours	Itraconazole, voriconazole
Every 24 hours	Fluconazole

Table XX. Frequency of administration of some time-dependent antifungal agents.

Frequency of administration	Antifungal agents
Every 24 hours	Amphotericin B, caspofungin, micafungin

Table XXI. Frequency of administration of some concentration-dependent antifungal agents.

8 CONCLUSIONS

In conclusion, the hope is that the goal of making easier the understanding of the principles underlying the movement of drugs within the body in relation to different pathophysiological or iatrogenic situations has been at least partially achieved, and that this publication may be useful to clinicians for the appropriate management of drug therapy in daily practice.

In a period like the current one, characterized by the gradual increase in life expectancy thanks to the availability of appropriate drug therapies for the treatment of many chronic diseases, it becomes essential to know how to properly handle the dosing regimens of drugs in relation to the patient's comorbidities and polytherapies, especially when the latter involve the use of many different drug classes.

In this regard, the knowledge of the principles of the pharmacokinetics, which is often considered as a specialistic science whose application essentially based on mathematical models is to be reserved to insiders only (the pharmacokineticists), can be of paramount relevance for the correct application of the valuable Hippocratic precept *primum non nocere*.

REFERENCES

- Andes D. In vivo pharmacodynamics of antifungal drugs in treatment of candidiasis. *Antimicrob Agents Chemother* 2003; 47: 1179-86
- Balayssac D, Authier N, Cayre A, Coudore F. Does inhibition of P-glycoprotein lead to drug-drug interactions? *Toxicol Lett* 2005; 156: 319-29
- Bartelink IH, Rademaker CM, Schobben AF, van den Anker JN. Guidelines on paediatric dosing on the basis of developmental physiology and pharmacokinetic considerations. *Clin Pharmacokinet* 2006; 45: 1077-97
- Bowden R, Chandrasekar P, White MH, Li X, Pietrelli L, Gurwith M, et al. A double-blind, randomized, controlled trial of amphotericin B colloidal dispersion versus amphotericin B for treatment of invasive aspergillosis in immunocompromised patients. *Clin Infect Dis* 2002; 35: 359-66
- Cotreau MM, von Moltke LL, Greenblatt DJ. The influence of age and sex on the clearance of cytochrome P450 3A substrates. *Clin Pharmacokinet* 2005; 44: 33-60
- Cusack BJ. Pharmacokinetics in older persons. *Am J Geriatr Pharmacother* 2004; 2: 274-302
- Delco F, Tchambaz L, Schlienger R, Drewe J, Krahenbuhl S. Dose adjustment in patients with liver disease. *Drug Saf* 2005; 28: 529-45
- DeRyke CA, Lee SY, Kuti JL, Nicolau DP. Optimising dosing strategies of antibacterials utilising pharmacodynamic principles: impact on the development of resistance. *Drugs* 2006; 66: 1-14

- Desta Z, Zhao X, Shin JG, Flockhart DA. Clinical significance of the cytochrome P450 2C19 genetic polymorphism. *Clin Pharmacokinet* 2002; 41: 913-58
- DuBuske LM. The role of P-glycoprotein and organic anion-transporting polypeptides in drug interactions. *Drug Saf* 2005; 28: 789-801
- Gardiner SJ, Begg EJ. Pharmacogenetics, drug-metabolizing enzymes, and clinical practice. *Pharmacol Rev* 2006; 58: 521-90
- Harris RZ, Jang GR, Tsunoda S. Dietary effects on drug metabolism and transport. *Clin Pharmacokinet* 2003; 42: 1071-88
- Mallet L, Spinewine A, Huang A. The challenge of managing drug interactions in elderly people. *Lancet* 2007; 370: 185-91
- McLean AJ, Le Couteur DG. Aging biology and geriatric clinical pharmacology. *Pharmacol Rev* 2004; 56: 163-84
- Meyer UA. Pharmacogenetics and adverse drug reactions. *Lancet* 2000; 356: 1667-71
- Munar MY, Singh H. Drug dosing adjustments in patients with chronic kidney disease. *Am Fam Physician* 2007; 75: 1487-96
- Pea F, Furlanut M. Pharmacokinetic aspects of treating infections in the intensive care unit: focus on drug interactions. *Clin Pharmacokinet* 2001; 40: 833-68
- Pea F, Russo D, Michieli M, Baraldo M, Ermacora A, Damiani D, et al. Liposomal daunorubicin plasmatic and renal disposition in patients with acute leukemia. *Cancer Chemother Pharmacol* 2000; 46: 279-86
- Pea F, Viale P. The antimicrobial therapy puzzle: could pharmacokinetic-pharmacodynamic relationships be helpful in addressing the issue of appropriate pneumonia treatment in critically ill patients? *Clin Infect Dis* 2006; 42: 1764-71

- Pea F, Viale P, Furlanut M. Antimicrobial therapy in critically ill patients: a review of pathophysiological conditions responsible for altered disposition and pharmacokinetic variability. *Clin Pharmacokinet* 2005; 44: 1009-34
- Scaglione F, Paraboni L. Influence of pharmacokinetics/pharmacodynamics of antibacterials in their dosing regimen selection. *Expert Rev Anti Infect Ther* 2006; 4: 479-90
- Schwartz JB. The current state of knowledge on age, sex, and their interactions on clinical pharmacology. *Clin Pharmacol Ther* 2007; 82: 87-96
- Smith SV, Gould IM. Optimization of antibiotic dosing schedules in the light of increasing antibiotic resistance. *Expert Rev Anti Infect Ther* 2004; 2: 227-34
- Spinewine A, Schmader KE, Barber N, Hughes C, Lapane KL, Swine C, et al. Appropriate prescribing in elderly people: how well can it be measured and optimised? *Lancet* 2007; 370: 173-84
- Turnheim K. Pharmacokinetic dosage guidelines for elderly subjects. *Expert Opin Drug Metab Toxicol* 2005; 1: 33-48
- Weinshilboum R. Inheritance and drug response. *N Engl J Med* 2003; 348: 529-37
- Whitten DL, Myers SP, Hawrelak JA, Wohlmuth H. The effect of St John's wort extracts on CYP3A: a systematic review of prospective clinical trials. *Br J Clin Pharmacol* 2006; 62: 512-26

GLOSSARY

Absorption

Process by which a drug reaches the systemic circulation.

Area under the plasma concentration-time curve (AUC)

Pharmacokinetic parameter that gives information on the extent of plasma drug exposure.

Compliance

The extent to which a person's behavior coincides with medical care or advice, for example, drug dosing regimens.

Cytochrome P450 (CYP)

Hepatic microsomal enzymatic system responsible for oxidative-reductive drug metabolism.

Distribution

Diffusion process of the drug from the blood to the tissues.

Dose finding

Studies carried out to evaluate the profile of plasma concentrations over time in relation to increasing doses of medication with the aim to determine the type of kinetics and the routes of elimination.

Elimination

Removal of the drug from the body through metabolism and/or excretion.

Enzyme

Protein that allows or accelerates a chemical or a biological reaction without being itself changed by the reaction.

Enzyme inducer

A substance able to promote the genetically predetermined production of enzymes, thus increasing their metabolic activity.

Enzyme inhibitor

A substance which binds to the enzymes, thus blocking their metabolic activity, reversibly or irreversibly.

Excretion

Process of elimination of a drug through the urine, the bile, etc.

First-pass effect

Pre-systemic metabolic degradation that occurs during the passage through the intestinal wall and/or the portal circulation and the liver.

Loading dose (LD)

The dose of medication always larger than the subsequent ones that is administered at the beginning of therapy with the purpose of filling rapidly the V_d occupied by the drug.

Maintenance dose (MD)

Dose that allows the maintenance of the therapeutically effective concentrations of the drug previously achieved by administering the LD.

Metabolism

Process of biotransformation of a drug, including phase I reactions (nonsynthetic) and phase II reactions (synthetic).

Oral bioavailability (F_{os})

The fraction of a drug (F) which, after administration by a route different from the intravenous one, reaches the systemic circulation in unchanged form (i.e., therapeutically active form), and the rapidity with which it does so.

P170 glycoprotein (Pgp)

Transmembrane protein normally present in many human cells that acts as a protective and detoxifying extrusive pump against many xenobiotics.

Pharmacodynamics

The science that studies the mechanism of action of drugs.

Pharmacokinetics

The science that studies the movement of drugs within a living organism.

Phase I reaction

Chemical reaction of enzymatic biotransformation that changes a drug into a more polar metabolite by oxidation, reduction, or hydrolysis.

Phase II reaction

Chemical reaction of enzymatic biotransformation that causes a bind between the drug, or its metabolites, with an endogenous substrate, such as glucuronic acid, sulfonates, acetic acid or aminoacids.

Plasma clearance (CL)

The volume of plasma that is cleared by the drug in the unit of time.

Plasma elimination half-life ($t_{1/2}$)

The time required for the amount of a substance to decrease by a half.

Prodrugs

Drugs that require metabolic activation into an active metabolite, in order to be effective.

Sequential therapy

Possibility of treating patients with the same drug sequentially by different routes of administration (usually before by IV and subsequently per os), according to the severity of the disease, but with the intent of ensuring equal therapeutic efficacy.

Steady state concentration (C_{ss})

Stable concentration which is reached and then maintained unchanged in the body when an equilibrium between the **inputs**, i.e., the doses of drug administered, and the **outputs**, i.e., the amount of drug that is eliminated by the excretory organs, has been achieved.

Time to reach steady state (t_{ss})

Time needed to reach the steady state.

Volume of distribution (V_d)

Also known as "apparent volume of distribution", it is the volume that the drug would occupy in the body if it had in all the body districts the same concentration that it has in plasma at time 0 after administration by intravenous bolus injection.

Xenobiotic

Substance which is found in the organism, but which is not normally present in it.

AUTHOR

Federico Pea

Medical Doctor in charge of Chemotherapy at the Institute of Clinical Pharmacology of the University Hospital of Udine, Italy, and contract professor at the post-graduate School of Clinical Pharmacology at the University of Udine, Italy.

Co-author of over 90 articles published in international peer-reviewed scientific journals with Impact Factor on topics of clinical pharmacology, antimicrobial and antineoplastic chemotherapy.

Member of the International Editorial Board of *Clinical Pharmacokinetics* and of *Pharmaceutics*, and reviewer for several other international scientific journals in various fields of clinical pharmacology and of antimicrobial chemotherapy.